# THE Qi OF
## Taking a
## Medical History
### — AND —
# Performing
# a Physical
# Examination

FRANK SEINSHEIMER III, M.D.

# APOLOGIA

During the writing of this book I was informed that my cancer has spread. I have an aggressive cancer which responds poorly to chemotherapy. As a direct result of this news, I accelerated my writing and my editing. I planned to use more vignettes, submitted by my colleagues, in medical fields other than my own. I, unfortunately, do not have time for that. Normally, as I write over many months, ideas pop into my consciousness without summoning. The shortened time period of writing means that there is less time for my brain to work subconsciously. Thus, there will be fewer epiphanies and fewer vignettes than I desire in this book. My normal editing process includes setting my manuscript aside for a few months and then rereading, rewriting and reediting. I do not have time for that. My writing, my organization, my thoughts will not be up to my own personal standards. Certainly, the editing will be sloppier and less thorough than I wish. For all of these defects, I apologize. Please understand my need for urgency.

Learn from everyone
Question everything
Decide for yourself
Become your own teacher

rambling permutations[1]
of synaptic excess
quantum fluctuations
of quarkian nonsense


irreducible conundrums
googleplexian math
quasilogical statements
circular boolean path

1    Poetical Commentary, Third Edition, Frank Seinsheimer III, Xlibris, 2015, Gibberwishy, page 105, lines 39-47

# TABLE OF CONTENTS

# CHAPTER ONE:

# Rambling Permutations of Synaptic Excess

Who am I writing this book for? Who is my audience? Why am I writing this book? What is the meaning of life? Just kidding. I am writing this book for medical students, nurse practitioner students, physician assistant students and others embarking on their exhilarating and intimidating journey into the terra incognito jungle of the clinical practice of medicine.

Prior to entering the life of clinical medical training, my educational life consisted of the traditional lecture, read, memorize; lecture, read, memorize; lecture, read, memorize, then finally try to understand approach to education. Entering my clinical training, I was stunned by the transition to the random apprenticeship method of clinical teaching. Astounded, dumbfounded, stupefied and startled are other synonymatic adjectives which round out my description of my reaction to my entry into the "practice" of clinical medicine.

Clinical medical training is remarkably and profoundly apprentice-like. In elementary school, in high school, in college and in the first two years of medical school my courses were taught within a logical framework in which the flow of knowledge ran from beginning concepts through intermediate concepts to more complex concepts. This seemingly logical method of instruction was the only method of instruction I had experienced throughout my formal educational career.

When I began my actual medical clinical training, the method of training, the method of education, the method of instruction changed drastically. I entered a random realm in which my learning depended on whichever patients, happenstance sent my way. I entered a seemingly accidental and arbitrary method of instruction, in which my learning depended on whichever mentors, teachers and patients, Tyche, the Greek goddess of chance, the capricious dispenser of good and ill fortune, placed in my meandering, seemingly drunken walk, life path.

I wish in this book to discuss in broad, sweeping strokes some basic concepts and some basic precepts inherent in the "proper" practice of taking a medical history and the "proper" practice of performing a medical physical examination. I wish to provide you with an understanding and a philosophical and psychological approach to your interactions with patients. I wish to provide you with some sense of an outline and advice in how to structure and perform your patient history taking and your patient physical examinations.

You will learn about history taking and physical examination performance far more from hands on experience than from didactic presentations. History taking and physical examination performance are not activities you have ever done before. If you are anything like me, you will find taking an excellent medical history and performing and excellent physical examination difficult, bewildering, frustrating and overwhelming at the start.

First, you need to know about the multitude of possible disease processes you may see in the patients, you encounter and you don't yet know them. Second, you need to know the myriad ways this multitude of disease processes cause symptoms and present as physical examination abnormalities. You will need to learn the multitude of ways sociological and psychological factors intermingle and intertwine with biological processes. This learning is a life-long process of which your medical school years are only the beginning. In the initial years of your clinical training you will form habits which will be lifelong.

**My purpose in writing this book is to nudge you toward forming good history taking habits and good physical examination performing habits early in your clinical career.**

This book differs from other instruction manuals which discuss the art of medical history taking and the science of performing a physical examination or is it the science of medical history taking and the art of performing a physical examination? In this book, I insert a multitude of case studies to illustrate my points. Many of these case studies involve physician errors which occurred due to either inadequate history taking or inadequate physical examinations. All of these case studies are true. None are fabricated. I repeat. All of these case studies are true. None are fabricated. The medical histories and the physical examinations, I present, were often deficient due to a failure to observe, evaluate and investigate with sufficient care and thought.

Yes!

I am harsh in my judgement. After all everyone makes mistakes.

But!

The consequences of mistakes in medicine are often life ending, life threatening or permanently life altering. Sadly. The mistakes of omission, the mistakes of missing something, the mistakes of failure to be thorough in medicine are common, common, common. Laziness, sloppy thinking and the lack of careful and thorough process are all too common.

Some of the case studies I present in this book involve experienced, clever, observant, aware, "On" clinicians who figured out obscure presentations quickly and seemingly effortlessly. In inserting these many case studies, I am attempting to teach you through second hand experience. Many of the cases are from my own personal experience. Other cases I have solicited from friends and colleagues. Because I am an orthopedic and hand surgeon many of my personal case studies come from those areas of medicine. The basic concepts are universal.

I have found over many years of practice that the extent of teaching of musculoskeletal medicine to non-orthopedic surgeon medical providers lies somewhere between inadequate and non-existent. Musculoskeletal problems are common. Patients with musculoskeletal problems are seen frequently by internists, general practice physicians, family medicine physicians, emergency room physicians, pediatricians, physician assistants and nurse practitioners. I have seen many missed diagnoses and inferior initial evaluations and treatment of medical and musculoskeletal problems over the years. These misses were at least partially the result of inadequate musculoskeletal medical training.

I hope in this book to offer sufficient musculoskeletal instruction to counter this lack. I shall include protocols or lists of what specifics I feel should be part of the history and physical examination of each part of the body. I shall provide frequent examples of patients for whom a limited history, a limited physical examination or more generally a limited overall evaluation led to inferior medical care. Inferior medical histories and inferior physical examinations by definition inevitably lead to inferior medical care.

What attitudes and behaviors create the difference between an average, so-so, ordinary, ho-hum, mundane physician or surgeon and an outstanding, excellent physician or surgeon? What is the difference between the truly competent physician and the rest of the pack? The difference lies in the excellent physician's attitude and approach to life, the universe and the practice of medicine and surgery.

Despite the near miraculous advances in medicine and surgery, taking a medical history and performing a physical examination remain the basic and fundamental underpinnings of the practice of medicine and surgery. In my interactions as a patient with specialist physicians, I find a remarkable decrease in the use of the physical examination and a remarkable decrease in the details of medical history taking.

Taking the medical history and performing the physical examination form the initial interaction between the medical provider and the patient in most cases. For many physicians taking the medical history and performing the physical examination seems a boring, rote exercise. For the excellent physician, taking the medical history and performing the physical examination is not haphazard. For the excellent physician, taking the medical history and performing the physical examination is the beginning of a planned, controlled investigation performed in a precise, orderly and thoughtful proceeding. The outstanding physician is constantly curious, looking for unexpected or hidden clues which will indicate a problem which is not immediately obvious. For the excellent physician, the medical history and physical examination is similar to a police detective procedural sniffing out the dog which didn't bark in the night.

The difference between the excellent, outstanding physician and the ordinary, average physician is attitude. When you take a medical history and perform a physical examination do you just go through rote motions?

OR.

Do you have a desperate desire to avoid missing something?

I have seen and personally experienced far too much ordinary medicine in my life.

SO.

Back to "Why am I writing this book?"

I am writing this book in an attempt to stimulate you to strive to improve and perfect your diagnostic abilities. I am writing this book to stimulate you to ascend to excellence in the practice of medicine. I am writing this book to encourage you to develop your curiosity, your attitude and your observational skills to help you on this journey.

Yes! I am being preachy.

Yes! My feelings are strong.

I offer no apology for my hectoring.

I have written this book as an introduction and a teaching aid for medical school students, general practice residents, family medicine residents, pediatric residents, emergency medicine residents, nurse practitioners, physician assistants, orthopedic residents and anyone else in the medical profession who wishes to expand their abilities in the evaluation and diagnosis of medical problems.

There is increasing specialization in all areas of medicine and surgery. Specialists often see their patients only through the narrow slit lens of their subspecialty. These specialists tend to ignore complaints which are not wedged into their increasingly small niche practice. Some super specialists will not even see a patient referral without an MRI. Their approach to medical history taking and physical examination may be perfunctory since they rely so heavily on scans.

Following medical school, I was a general surgery intern for one year and a general surgery junior resident for one year. I then spent one year in a research lab. During that year I moonlighted covering emergency rooms in suburban hospitals every fifth night. This occurred before specialists in emergency medicine were prevalent. I was the only physician present in those emergency rooms for my entire twelve hour shift. I spent three years in an orthopedic residency, two years as an orthopedic surgeon in the U. S. Army and then one year as a hand and microvascular fellow.

I practiced general orthopedics and hand surgery for 37 ½ years. I saw patients in the office 3 ½ days a week and operated 1 ½ days a week. During that time, I saw approximately 100 patient office visits each week. That averages out to about three and a half patients each hour. Multiply times 40 weeks (allowing for vacation and education time off) and I estimate I saw approximately 4000 patient office visits a year. Multiply that conservatively times 35 and I estimate I saw approximately 140,000 patient office visits in my career not counting my in-training patient encounters.

During those years of practice, I tried as much as possible to be the complete physician.

Here are the first two case studies. There are plenty more to come.

*Case Study:*
*A patient is referred to my office, an orthopedic surgeon's office, with a heel draining white, chalk-like material. Having seen this before, I immediately recognize this as classic chronic gout with a draining tophus. I probably saw ten draining gout tophi in my career. All involved either the feet or the fingers. In this case, I am able to immediately diagnose the draining tophus as gout. So, how much of a history do I need to take? I mean really, I have the diagnosis immediately. Besides, gout is a "medical" problem. Right. Just send the patient back to the internist. Right? What else is there to do?*

*I spend time taking his medical history. My patient gives a history of multiple previous episodes of gout attacks. I know from experience this usually means that the patient is refusing gout medication or is not taking his prescribed gout medication. The patient's uric acid blood level is elevated. It is surprising how many men refuse to take their gout medication due to some weird macho thing. I question my patient carefully regarding his gout medication. He swears that he takes his gout medicine regularly, as prescribed. While many patients lie to us, physicians, this patient seems earnest and truthful. My patient is Hispanic. I take the time to question him further using an interpreter.*

*I am intrigued by this mystery. I ask myself, "Why? Exactly why, is my patient having recurrent gout attacks?" Why is he showing evidence of chronic gout with a draining tophus in his heel despite taking his gout medicine regularly? Why does his uric acid level remain elevated? Is this some unusual, previously undescribed resistant gout syndrome?*

*Anyway, controlling gout is a medical problem. Right! Let the internist take care of it. Right!*

*NO!*

*I try to be a complete physician, when I can. I continue my medical history. I am curious. I want an answer. I want an explanation. Internally, I demand of myself that I find the answer. I take the time to question further. Finally, after many questions, I think to ask, "Where do you get your gout medication from?" He replies, "El Salvador, very cheap." Clearly, he is taking "fraudulent" medication. I advise him to obtain his gout medication from an American pharmacy. He does. His gout is then controlled.*

*Proper treatment for this patient required the time, the thought, the energy and the curiosity to recognize the fact that a "mystery" existed and then to solve the "mystery." Proper treatment for this patient required an extensive, thoughtful and thorough medical history in order to solve this problem. Fancy scans would* not have solved this problem. This patient had seen three other medical doctors who had not sorted out the reason this patient had "recalcitrant" gout which was resisting treatment.

This case is also an example of the interaction, intersection and intermingling between the biology of the patient and the sociology of the patient. Simply put, the act of diagnosing gout and the act of prescribing gout medication alone did not result in successful medical treatment. Thoughtful and detailed history taking was required for success.

Here is the second case study.

*Case Study:*
*A yoga teacher has felt chronically ill for several years. She has intermittent gastrointestinal symptoms. Her internists have questioned her regarding foreign travel. She has not travelled out of the country. Her internists have not found the cause of her symptoms. One of her yoga students is an epidemiologist who learns of the teacher's symptoms. The yoga student, epidemiologist, takes an abbreviated medical history from her yoga teacher. The yoga student learns that the yoga teacher takes a supplement twice a day. The yoga student, epidemiologist, asks for a sample of the supplement.*

*Evaluation of the supplement by the epidemiologist shows that it is loaded with live parasites. Yes! Live parasites! Egad! Yuk! Erk! Ugh! Imagine! This yoga teacher has been dosing herself with live parasites twice a day for years. Her internist and her gastrointestinal consultant did not consider the possibility of intestinal parasites because the yoga teacher denied foreign travel. The supplement was imported from a country in Asia. It took an epidemiologist, yoga student, to ask the right medical history questions and perform the right diagnostic test in order to successfully diagnose this patient's problem.*

If you don't take a sufficiently detailed medical history, if you don't figure out the right questions to ask, if you don't try hard enough, you may not solve a patient's *problem. For this particular patient, the internist and gastrointestinal consultants did not ask sufficiently detailed questions to solve this unusual problem.*

The two case studies described above demonstrate that the successful practice of medicine is not always fancy scans and sophisticated science. The two case studies described above demonstrate that the successful practice of medicine may involve subtle investigation. The excellent practice of medicine involves careful and thoughtful evaluations of your patients' problems. Not just ordering scans.

Let me again ask the question.

What is the difference between an average medical provider and an outstanding medical provider?

Please! Stop! Think about this question!

I will let you answer the question this time.

Let me ask another question.

Which of the two types of medical providers do you wish to be?

The outstanding medical provider will:

1.  Have a desperate desire to figure out the diagnosis or diagnoses and the causes of the diagnosis or diagnoses
2.  Constantly be on the lookout for problems outside of his/her specialty
3.  Be curious and always look for the unexpected and unusual
4.  Be observant for subtle cues and clues
5.  Be sufficiently obsessive and compulsive to minimize the chance of missing information and/or making a mistake
6.  Be able to communicate properly with patients, family and colleagues

I wish in this book to give you a sense of what is out there and what you may see. I wish to give you a sense of what you <u>may</u> miss if you are insufficiently curious. I wish to give you a sense of what you <u>may</u> miss if you are insufficiently careful. Let me restate that. I wish to give you a sense of what you <u>will</u> miss if you are insufficiently curious. I wish to give you a sense of what you <u>will</u> miss if you are insufficiently careful. I wish to emphasize that you will not know everything. I wish to emphasize that you should be open to recognizing that a patient may have a problem you know nothing about and have never seen before.

If you see forty patients a week for fifty weeks a year for a forty year career you will have had eighty thousand patient interactions in your career.

If you may be involved in 80,000 patient interactions in your career, pure random chance suggests that you will have a 50/50 chance of seeing in your practice one patient with every problem which occurs only once in 160,000 people. Will you be sufficiently curious and thoughtful to recognize these unusual presentations when these patients come to your office?

Many of the clinical examples which I use in this book have been discussed in my other medical book, my medical memoir, "The Qi of the Scalpel." I have repurposed these vignettes in this book for teaching purposes.

Note! I use many medical terms in this book without defining them. As students beginning your medical clinical training many of these medical terms may not be familiar to you. If I stop to define every medical term I use, I will double the size of this book and slow down the flow of information. As beginning students, I encourage you to look up each and every medical term you do not recognize. That will make reading this book even more educational.

My purpose in writing this book is to provide you with an attitude, an approach and an understanding of the importance of taking careful and thoughtful medical histories and performing careful and thoughtful physical examinations.

# CHAPTER TWO

# The Intersection between the medical history and the physical examination

## The importance of observation

A patient's medical history and physical examination are inseparably intermingled, intermixed and intertwined with each other. A patient's medical history informs the medical provider's presumptive differential diagnosis or diagnoses prior to the physical examination. The patient's medical history informs the examining medical provider what type of physical examination is appropriate. In order to take a proper patient history and perform a proper physical examination, the diagnosing medical provider needs to have knowledge of the possible diagnoses and their manifestations in the physical examination.

Actually, the patient's physical examination usually begins before the medical history taking begins. Why? Because the physician is already observing and evaluating the patient before beginning to take the medical history.

One critical aspect of any physical examination is observation. Many of us go through our lives observing little of the world around us. The next time you drive up to a red traffic light and are slowing down to stop, look at the people crossing in the crosswalk in front of you. Most of them are looking straight ahead or down at the ground. Only rarely do you see one of the pedestrians turn her head and look at you and your car to see if you are actually slowing down to stop. Most pedestrians are not alert. Most pedestrians are not aware of the world around them. Most pedestrians are focused inward on themselves. To generalize: Most people are not alert. Most people are not aware of the world around them. Most people are focused inward on themselves.

When I was in college I took a course on social psychology. I recall learning about a study that touches on the subject of observation. The investigators went into a prison and showed movies of people walking down the street to convicted muggers. This was before the days of video and computers.

The convicted predators were asked to identify which people walking down the street they might attack and which they would avoid attacking. The people walking down the street looking at the ground and obviously unaware of the world around them were identified as possible prey. The people walking with their heads up, looking around and obviously aware of their surroundings were identified as people to avoid.

Which type of person walking down the street are you?

I encourage you to expand your observation of the world around you.

Look at people.

Observe them.

Coincident with expanding your observation of the world around you, you want to expand your observation of your patients. Depending on the situation you may first see your next patient walking down the hall, in an exam room sitting in a chair or lying on a bed or gurney.

What do you see at first glance? How is the patient dressed? What clothing is the patient wearing? What job might they have? Does the patient seem alert or have a vacant look?

"From one thing, know ten thousand things."

This quote from Miyamoto Murashi's "The Book of Five Rings" emphasizes the attitude, the approach and the philosophy of intense, careful and thoughtful observation and intense, careful and thoughtful analysis of that observation. Miyamoto Murashi was a famed Japanese duelist and undefeated samurai who wrote this book in 1643 after retiring having won approximately fifty duels.

Here are some case studies that deal with the "observation" theme.

*Case Study:*
*I walk into an exam room to see a new orthopedic patient. I have glanced at the chart. He has good insurance. Yet, he and his clothes are dirty, disheveled and smelly. My immediate "observation" is the dichotomy between his excellent insurance coverage and his demeanor, appearance and odor, yes odor. The immediate response of many physicians would be to get rid of the patient as quickly as possible and refer the patient to the local free clinic.*

*And. Yet! And. Yet! And. Yet!*

*I am intrigued by the dichotomy mentioned above. Mental illness and/or homelessness are certainly possible explanations. Yet, he looks alert and looks at me with his eyes in an apparent thoughtful manner. How should I begin taking this patient's medical history? For the first question, I ask about this dichotomy. I* say, "I'm confused. You have excellent medical insurance, but you don't look like someone with excellent medical insurance. What is going on?" The dichotomy is quickly solved. He is an undercover police officer, who is really good at what he does. He has come to my office directly from work.

Note my use of the general question "What is going on?" General, open ended questions are often a great way to start a medical history.

*Case Study:*
*I am working in the gynecology clinic of a major medical center and see a patient with the common complaint of vaginal bleeding. My patient tells me that she noticed the bleeding this morning when she awoke. She says the bleeding started spontaneously. On vaginal examination, I observe unusual, extensive abrasions up and down the walls of her vagina. Startled by this unusual finding, which I have never seen before, I continue my medical history using a broad, general question, "What's been going on?" She tells me that she had sex with multiple partners the previous night. The cause of the abnormal physical examination observation is solved with a single general question?*

I present the next two cases more for humor than any real teaching point. These cases demonstrate the benefit of careful observation. These stories are true.

*Case Study:*
*I am called to the Greater Laurel Beltsville Hospital emergency room to see a woman in her 30s who has broken her wrist. As I walk toward her bed, I notice that her home address is in the Laurel area but her insurance guarantor is the Australian embassy. My first medical history question is, "Why do you live out in Laurel if you work at the Australian embassy." She replies, "My husband works at Fort Meade." I reply, "He must work at the National Security Agency." She replies, "I can't tell you that." I treat her wrist fracture.*

*Two weeks later, I am called to the Greater Laurel Beltsville Hospital emergency room to see a man in his early 30s with an injured ankle. I notice that his home address is different from the case above, but also in the Laurel area. I note that his insurance guarantor is also the Australian embassy. I walk up to his stretcher, smile, introduce myself and shake his hand. I say, "You must be one the Australians working at the National Security Agency." The look of shock and surprise on his face was one I have never seen before or since. I have read about the expression "his jaw dropped in surprise." This is the only time in my life I actually saw it happen. After a minute or two of gasping and sputtering, he asks, "Does everyone know?"*

In the practice of medicine, only with proper observation and thought can you have this much fun!

Observation of the patient begins at the first sight or hearing of the patient. Why do I mention hearing?

*Case Study:*

*I am sitting in a center city emergency room writing in a patient's chart. This was before the advent of electronic medical records. I hear an ambulance with sirens blaring pull up. Moments later, a patient in wheeled into the emergency room, on a stretcher screaming and shouting at the maximum decibels any human is capable of reaching. I do not see the patient since the patient is around a corner. What is my immediate observation? Probably not an acute emergency? Why? It requires tremendous effort, tremendous cardiac function, tremendous respiratory function and fully functioning neurologic function to scream that loud continually. The patients who lie still and are not moving are of greater concern.*

*Case Study:*

*I am walking through the emergency room with three fellow first year medical students and our mentor, Dr. Alan Birtch, at the Peter Bent Brigham Hospital. We are in our first month of medical school. We stop to talk to an elderly woman with a grossly swollen, deformed right wrist. Dr. Birtch is showing us what an* emergency room is and how it is structured. As untrained and as clueless as I am medically at that time, even I am able to observe that this woman clearly has an acute fracture of the right wrist. The right wrist is grossly deformed and swollen.

To my surprise, Dr. Birtch asks the patient when she broke her other wrist. There is a subtle deformity of the other wrist. None of us early first year medical students noticed this subtle deformity. Our mentor did. This is the "immediate," "first impression," "careful observation" part of the physical exam, in action.

This vignette was my first medical clinical training epiphany. I recognized that I needed to expand my observation and awareness skills. Some fifty four years later, this vignette remains indelibly fixed and vivid in my memory.

Why might it be important to recognize that this patient has had previous falls and fractures. Further evaluation should include searching for the multiple causes of recurrent falls and evaluating for probable osteoporosis. Further treatment might include intervening to try to minimize the risk of falls in the future as well as possible treatment of osteoporosis. Failure to observe the subtle deformity of the other wrist and/or failure to inquire about previous falls and/or fractures would lead to a failure to diagnose and treat the cause of the falls and the osteoporosis.

Case Study

A high school friend of mine flew home from college on vacation. He walked to meet his family at the airport. His mother, not a physician, noted that my friend was jittery as he approached. My friend also had bulging eyes. My friend's mother immediately said to my friend, "You have an overactive thyroid. I taking you right over to our doctor." An excellent expert immediate observation diagnosis by a non-physician.

17

What is a patient's history? How do you take a history from a patient or family member? A patient's history is the information you obtain from the patient or family member about the reason the patient is seeing a physician. The history should also include anything else and everything else which might impact this patient's health and wellbeing.

Obviously, some histories are straight forward. For example: "I missed a step and turned my ankle. I can't walk on it. My ankle is swollen. My ankle hurts" Short, concise, pithy, to the point. What else is needed in this medical history? Just move on to the physical exam and x-ray.

Right? Right?

And. Yet! And. Yet! And. Yet!

Why did the patient trip, fall and injure his ankle? What are the possibilities? Let's make a list: the most likely possibility, of course, is ordinary, momentary inattention while walking. Other possibilities include: a physical attack and the patient does not wish to admit that; abuse by a boyfriend, girlfriend, husband or wife; failing vision; drug use; early neurologic deterioration of numerous types including multiple sclerosis, adult onset muscular dystrophies; peripheral neuropathies; neurosyphilis; brain tumor; petit mal seizure and on and on and on. I can fill a multi-volume textbook discussing possible non-standard, non-common reasons a patient may "stumble and injure an ankle."

Even in an apparently simple, straightforward case of a sprained or broken ankle, the observant, questioning physician will look for additional causes, additional diagnoses and additional issues which should be evaluated for possible intervention.

Am I overstating the case?

*Case Study:*

*A forty two year old man comes into my office with the complaint of ankle pain. He states that he twisted his ankle three and a half weeks ago. He saw another orthopedic surgeon who gave him an ankle brace. He returned to see the orthopedic surgeon after three weeks complaining of increasing ankle pain. The orthopedic surgeon, by the patient's history, jerked on the ankle and accused the patient of being lazy and not wanting to work. This patient might have gone to his internist or family practitioner or to an emergency room for this second visit. The other orthopedic surgeon was Caucasian. The patient was Black. The patient was an engineer. The patient came to my office a few days after the second office visit with the original orthopedic surgeon.*

*So, is this a histrionic and/or faking and/or lazy patient? Is this patient shirking work?*

*My office was packed that day. I was running behind. This patient was placed in our cast room by my assistant given the apparent diagnosis of ankle sprain. As I took the above history from the patient, I noted that the swelling about the ankle was globular in shape. The swelling was not the shape I would expect from a chronic, abused sprained ankle. The x-rays in the first orthopedic surgeon's office were negative except for some soft tissue swelling on both sides of the ankle. I believed the patient. The ankle looked more swollen and in a different shape than I would expect from a three and a half week old abused sprain.*

*Here is where the patient's medical history and the physical examination intermingle, intertwine, intersect. They mutually influence each other. The patient's history helps inform what physical examination to perform. The physical examination informs what further history to obtain. In this case the combination of the initial history and the observational initial physical examination informed the need for and the direction of my further medical history taking. So far, the physical examination has just been observation as the patient and I sit across from each other.*

*My immediate observational differential diagnosis includes inflammatory arthritis, infectious arthritis as well as overuse and abuse of a sprained ankle. Of these possible diagnoses, determining the possibility of an infectious arthritis takes precedence. Missing the diagnosis of infectious arthritis, if the diagnosis is correct, will lead to harm to the patient.*

*With this in mind, I start to take the patient's history. This is a true story. My first question: "Have you had unprotected sex in the past three to four months?" Why this question? Gonorrheal septic arthritis can present with a swollen joint in the absence of symptoms or complaints in the genital region. The gonorrhea bacteria may lay dormant for months before causing symptoms. I personally have seen a number of cases of septic gonorrheal arthritis of the wrist, ankle and hip. All gave a positive medical history of unprotected sex in the previous four months. Based on the globular swelling of the ankle, gonorrheal septic arthritis is immediately high on my differential diagnosis list. An uncommon diagnosis? Yes. But. An uncommon looking ankle, despite the "normal" medical history. My patient's answer to my first question, "Yes."*

*My second question, "Heterosexual or homosexual?" His answer, "Homosexual." I asked this question because we were in the early days of the AIDS epidemic. The patient's positive answer to my second question resulted in my adding AIDS to my differential diagnosis list. After further evaluation, I transferred my patient that afternoon to the hospital and performed ankle arthroscopy to wash out the joint and to obtain good cultures for identification of the bacteria causing the infection and for bacterial sensitivities to antibiotics. Cultures showed gonococcus. Blood tests for HIV were positive. He was in a long term committed relationship. Unknown to him, unfortunately, his partner was having unprotected sexual contacts outside of his relationship with my patient.*

*This was a case of a "simple" ankle sprain which was NOT a "simple" ankle sprain. The initial "observation" led me quickly to three diagnoses. What were the three diagnoses? Healing sprained ankle, gonorrheal septic arthritis of the ankle joint and HIV infection.*

*Note my use of the word, "diagnoses." You never want to laser focus on one diagnosis only. You always want to look for more than one diagnosis. Simply put, the other orthopedic surgeon remained focused only on the obvious sprained ankle and did not consider other diagnoses. In other words, the other orthopedic surgeon blew it.*

*Needless to say, after finishing my evaluation of this complicated patient, scheduling the emergency surgery and calling for an infectious disease consult, I was even further behind in my clinic.*

As I stated in the preface, I am going to insert vignettes which I hope will provide practical examples to illustrate my teaching points. I hope the insertion of these actual clinical experiences serves to highlight and emphasize my teaching points. By using these vignettes, I am trying to give you, in a second hand way, additional clinical experience to assist your training.

*Case Study:*
*This is a true story. A teenage boy comes to my office complaining of an ankle sprain. Yep. Another simple, straight forward ankle sprain. The ankle is swollen on the lateral side of the lateral malleolus and looks like an ordinary ankle sprain with tearing of the lateral collateral ligaments. Do I simply splint the ankle and ask him to return in three weeks? OR, do I look for other diagnoses?*

*One important question to ask any patient with an ankle sprain, "Have you sprained this ankle before?" I ask this question. I am looking for the possibility of recurrent ankle sprains. He replies, "Yes, I have sprained this ankle five times before." One question; one answer. Suddenly, my differential diagnosis list expands. A history of five ankle sprains in a teenage boy is a statistical outlier. You will find that I use the phrase, "statistical outlier" frequently. I am constantly looking for patients who in some way are "statistical outliers" worthy of more detailed evaluation.*

*This initial medical history of now six ankle sprains cries for further evaluation. My differential diagnosis now includes chronic lateral ligament instability from complete rupture of the lateral ankle ligaments. My differential diagnosis also includes Ehlers-Danlos syndrome, a problem with congenital laxity of soft tissue including ligaments. As part of my physical exam I look to see if his thumb will touch the surface of the volar forearm. It does easily. If the tip of the thumb easily touches the volar forearm when the wrist is fully volar flexed, this simply indicates general ligament laxity. Alone, this finding does not specifically indicate a diagnosis of Ehlers-Danlos syndrome.*

*I continue my physical examination looking for evidence of Ehlers-Danlos syndrome. I find excessive laxity of many joints. I then look for unusual skin laxity and find it. I treat the ankle sprain and refer him for genetic work up to find out which form of Ehlers-Danlos syndrome he has, so that he can be counseled and followed up for this diagnosis.*

*One of the many reasons making this diagnosis is important is the fact that these patients do poorly, really poorly, really, really poorly after any ligament reconstruction surgery. Knowledge of this diagnosis is important for planning treatment of his ankle ligament instability. Surgery to repair his chronic ligament instability is guaranteed to fail. Treatment involves long term brace protection. The previous orthopedic surgeons who treated sprains number two through four did not ask after previous sprains and did not assess for Ehlers-Danlos syndrome. Plainly speaking, they missed the more important diagnosis. I estimate that I made the diagnosis of Ehlers-Danlos syndrome about five times in my career. There are more than ten types of Ehlers-Danlos syndrome described in the world literature. Some are mild with subtle findings. You need to be looking for this diagnosis to find it when the findings are subtle.*

I recall attending a hand surgery symposium years ago. At one of the afternoon sessions, the presenting hand surgeons were asked to present one of the more difficult cases in their career. One hand surgeon presented the case of a patient who underwent six operations with failed results before the diagnosis of Ehlers-Danlos syndrome was "realized." A hand surgeon with a world-wide reputation who quite simply missed the diagnosis of Ehlers-Danlos syndrome in a patient of his despite years of failed surgeries. A great lesson for the attendees of the hand surgery symposium. This world renowned hand surgeon had missed this diagnosis over many years of treatment involving multiple failed surgeries. I appreciate his integrity in presenting this case to us as a cautionary tale.

Obviously, most ankle sprains will be simple, ordinary, garden variety, minor ligament tears to the ankle. BUT! I REPEAT, BUT! NOT, ALL! You need to constantly look for the unexpected, the unusual, the statistical outlier. You need to have your nose to the wind and your antennae quivering and sensitive, constantly searching for the subtle clue or cue that you need to investigate further. Both of the case studies described above came into my office as "routine" ankle sprain cases. Both of these patients had seen at least one other orthopedic surgeon. As described, these cases were not routine ankle sprain cases. Careful and thoughtful observation and careful and thoughtful history taking were the behaviors necessary in the successful evaluations at these patient's first office visits.

*Case Study:*
*I am called to the emergency room to see a patient with a dislocated shoulder which the emergency room physician is unable to reduce back into the joint. The patient gives a history of falling off of the back of a truck and injuring his shoulder. Examination shows a prominent humeral head anteriorly. X-rays showed a "routine" anterior dislocation of the shoulder. I attempt closed reduction in the emergency room under sedation and am unsuccessful. I take him to the operating room. I attempt closed reduction under general anesthesia which always works. Well, always works, except when it doesn't. Unsuccessful. I assume this is a rare case of irreducible anterior dislocation of the shoulder, I open the shoulder joint surgically.*

*I find the humeral head anterior to the shoulder joint. The volume of the shoulder joint is filled with old scar. There is no bleeding and no evidence of a new injury. This is clearly a case of an "old" and neglected anterior dislocation of the shoulder. I close the surgical wound.*

*As I analyze this case some 40 years later, I think that I failed to ask this patient the important question, "Have you ever injured this shoulder before?" Had I asked that question, I likely would have prevented the unnecessary trip to the operating room. I was in my first year or two of practice. I was still learning. This was the case that cemented in my brain the need to ask detailed past history questions early and often. Why did I fail to ask the question about previous injuries to the shoulder? I think I was fooled by the presentation of a seemingly obvious acute anterior dislocation of the shoulder.*

*Case Study:*
*Another "simple" injury. A ten year old boy is running. He falls and hits his knee on a hard surface. The knee swells. Dad brings him in for a "routine" knee injury, orthopedic office visit. He might have come to the office of any general medical provider. The patient's clinical history is otherwise negative. He feels fine. Physical examination (which we will get to later in this book) shows an effusion (excess fluid) in the knee joint. There is no bruising. No black and blue. No superficial evidence of a contusion. No scrape. No abrasion of the skin. Other than the swelling from the joint effusion, the knee is normal on physical examination.*

*It is unusual for an external blow to cause an effusion in a joint with no other evidence of injury to the skin or soft tissue. Let me restate that, I think it is impossible for an external blow to an extremity to cause an effusion in a joint with no other evidence of injury to the skin or soft tissue. In fact, I have never seen it. Thus, I recognize the fact that this case is another statistical outlier. The history of the injury and the physical examination presentation are incompatible. The medical history is negative for fever or arthritic symptoms. With the absence of any skin or soft tissue evidence of injury, I suspect some spontaneous inflammation of the joint, either arthritic or infectious in nature. I suspect that the history of the injury is not the cause of this patient's presentation. The lack of significant pain and tenderness suggests that this is not a serious bacterial joint sepsis which requires urgent treatment.*

*I order blood work including a Lyme titer to test for Lyme disease. Lyme disease is endemic in Maryland where I am practicing. One week later, the test comes back positive for Lyme disease. I call Mom. Mom tells me that the swelling and the fluid in the knee have gone away. Her son is fine. I get an attitude of "Why are you bothering me?" I inform her of the positive Lyme test and refer her son to an infectious disease specialist for proper antibiotic treatment.*

*Yes, most closed contusion injuries to the knee are minor and self healing. The presence of the effusion when there should not have been an effusion pushed me to aggressively evaluate this patient at the first office visit with proper blood work. Early treatment of Lyme disease decreases the risk of chronic Lyme disease symptoms. Here, a "simple" contusion of the knee was not a "simple" contusion of the knee. Had I not been aggressive in ordering lab work at the first visit, the diagnosis would not have been made until later symptoms occurred.*

I present the preceding case studies to emphasize to you to the fact that you need to be constantly aware when evaluating patients. You need to constantly observe, assess and inquire. You need to follow up any subtle issues that arise. When you are busy, rushed and tired, it is easy to brush aside subtle signs, clues and cues. When you are being evaluated by the medical records system for how quickly you are seeing patients, it is easy to brush aside subtle signs, clues and cues. Following up subtle signs takes time. Following up subtle signs takes energy. Following up subtle signs takes curiosity. Following up subtle signs takes initiative. Many physicians fail in this task.

*Case Study:*
*I am called to the emergency room to see a 92 year old woman with a complex, displaced fracture of her finger. She slipped on icy steps coming out of church. I*

*take a detailed medical history including asking after history of heart attacks, chest pain, shortness of breath, etc. She replies, "No, No, No" to all. I take her to the operating room to fix her fracture. The anesthesiologist and I choose a Bier Block which is a safe, low stress method of arm anesthesia. Simply put, the arm is exsanguinated and the blood is temporarily replaced with local anesthetic and held in place with a pneumatic tourniquet.*

*The surgery is proceeding smoothly, when my patient begins to complain of crushing chest pain. Her EKG monitors show the classic changes for an acute myocardial infarction. Fortunately, my patient remains stable. After surgery is completed, she is transferred to the ICU and to the care of cardiologists.*

*The next morning on rounds I tell her that I am surprised she had a heart attack during surgery considering that she had never had any symptoms of heart trouble before. My patient laughs and says, "Oh doctor, I have been having chest pains for a week." I replied, "If you were having chest pains for a week, why didn't you tell me?" Her priceless reply, "Oh doctor, I didn't want to worry you." I present this vignette to emphasize the point that patients will not always tell you the truth. They will not always tell you the truth even if their motives are "good."*

Performing a complete patient history and physical examination involves mentally considering and mentally listing in your mind the differential diagnoses. What is the differential diagnosis? The differential diagnosis is your provisional list of probable diagnoses (causes) of the patient's symptoms. The moment you begin to interact with a patient, you immediately begin to list possible diagnoses in your head. You place the most likely diagnoses at the top of the list. Any diagnoses, which may not be likely, but which would be important to know early, such as an infection, should be at the top of the list also.

As you gain more information through asking questions, through observing the patient and through your physical examination, you alter your provisional list of probable diagnoses depending on the information gained. You shift your questions and you shift your physical examination as your interaction with the patient proceeds. Over time your differential diagnosis or diagnoses changes as you receive various test results.

It is important to constantly look for more than one diagnosis.

*Case Study:*
*A 45 year old man presents in my office with complaints of right shoulder pain following a fall while skiing. He is unable to actively lift his right arm against gravity. This patient has an obvious large rotator cuff tear of his right shoulder which likely will require surgery. Should I stop my evaluation and schedule physical therapy and surgery?*

*I ask additional questions. I try to be a complete physician. Rather than just focusing on the shoulder, I ask additional questions that are considered a review of systems. I do this for two reasons. One, the patient probably has a large rotator cuff tear of his shoulder which will require surgical correction. I need to know his general medical status to evaluate if he is a reasonable surgical candidate. I also routinely ask a quick review of systems, just trying to be a complete physician.*

*As part of my review of systems, I ask about numbness and tingling. My patient responds with elicited complaints of numbness and tingling of both upper extremities. I ask if he has more trouble opening tight jar lids than he used to. This is a good question looking for subtle upper extremity weakness. My patient replies, "Yes." Further questioning, discloses complaints of subtle weakness in both upper extremities.*

*Examination shows muscle atrophy in both hands in ulnar and median nerve innervated muscles with decreased light touch sensation. Further evaluation discloses the expected large rotator cuff tear of the shoulder on MRI which requires surgical correction. Further evaluation with electromyography documents severe bilateral carpal tunnel syndrome and severe bilateral cubital* tunnel syndrome of both arms with fasciculations in muscles innervated by both median nerves and both ulnar nerves. My patient needs bilateral carpal tunnel releases and bilateral cubital tunnel decompression surgery as well as the rotator cuff repair.

Patients frequently have more than one diagnosis. Finding five diagnoses requiring surgical correction at a first visit is obviously unusual. I present this case as an example of the importance of evaluating the "whole" patient, rather than laser focusing on the one presenting complaint.

**My point: Always evaluate the whole patient. Always look for additional diagnoses.**

# CHAPTER FOUR

# Ambiguity of language

---

## Superficial pain and deep pain

---

## Difficulty describing symptoms

---

## Symptoms may be caused by a problem outside of your specialty

---

## What kind of work do you do?

---

## How do you use your body?

---

Let's examine the "life history" of the taking of a patient's history. The patient's history is usually born with a complaint. I will ignore for the moment the issue of taking a history from others when the patient is unconscious or otherwise unable or unwilling to give a history. Sometimes the life cycle of a patient's history will begin with an observation.

As the patient answers questions, new issues may arise. The average physician will ignore some of the answers and just focus on the one problem which seems to be the focus of the patient's visit. This is faster and less complicated. The excellent physician will follow all of the faint trails which arise during the history and physical examination. Unexpected findings on the physical exam may lead to a pause and the need for additional history taking. Yes, there are occasional patients who will respond positively with complaints to any and every question. These patients need careful assessment. Even hypochondriacs can have real problems.

The medical history usually starts with a general question such as: "What can I do for you today?" or "What is the problem?" or "How are you doing today?" or "Tell me what's going on." or "What's up?" or "What brings you here today?"

For example, let's say a patient responds with "My shoulder hurts." The initial broad strokes differential diagnosis will include pain referred from the neck, a scapular problem or a problem with the shoulder joint area itself. The examining physician needs to be aware that there may be non-orthopedic causes of the problem.

What are some of the non-orthopedic problems which may present with the complaint of shoulder pain: myocardial infarction with radiation of pain to the left arm; shingles; Pancoast Syndrome which is the spread of a lung cancer into to brachial plexus nerves near the shoulder; irritation of the diaphragm may cause referred pain to the shoulder because the phrenic nerve derives from C3-5 and C4 and C5 innervate areas around the shoulder. The diaphragm may be irritated by biliary colic, liver abscess, ectopic pregnancy, pelvic inflammatory disease, subcostal abscess and intestinal perforation. The examining medical provider always needs to be aware that the cause of the chief complaint may be one of these "way out in left field" diagnoses.

The vertical part of the body under the head is obviously called the neck. The upper, outer corner of the thoracic area is obviously called the shoulder. What do we call the horizontal part of the body between the neck and the point of the shoulder? I don't know of any commonly used name for that part of the superficial anatomy. I have found that most patients who have pain in the horizontal part of the body between the neck and the point of the shoulder will complain of pain in the shoulder.

I always ask my patients to point to where the pain or discomfort hurts the most. Patients who point to the point of the shoulder most likely have a shoulder problem. Patients who point to the horizontal area between the neck and the shoulder more likely have pain from the neck or the scapula. Asking a patient where the pain or discomfort hurts the most is one of the most useful questions when taking a medical history from a patient complaining about pain or discomfort. This is not the last time I will emphasize this.

Other questions I ask are: "How long the shoulder has been bothering you?" "Please describe the pain? Where is the pain? Does it travel anywhere? Is it steady? Does it come and go?? If so, "How often do you get the pain" "What positions or activities seem to make the pain better or worse?" "Do you hurt anywhere else?" "Does anything else bother you?" "Have you had problems with this shoulder before?" "Have you had pain like this before?" "Have you injured your shoulder before?" What activities are you unable to do because of this pain? Does the pain interfere with your sleep?

Having asked your patient where the pain or discomfort is greatest, you will find a myriad of possible responses. There are patients who do not listen to the question. They are simply waiting for you to stop talking and then tell you whatever is on their mind. These patients need to be gently guided back to your questions.

Some patients will point to a specific location. Others will move their hand is a somewhat vague way over an area of the body. There are two types of pain systems in the body. The superficial or skin pain system has the characteristics of being sharp in nature and precisely localized. Recall the last time you had a paper cut. You knew precisely where you cut yourself and it hurt "sharply." It was a distinct, localized, painful, sharp, "ouch" feeling. This is the superficial or skin level pain system.

The other pain system is the deep pain system. This has the characteristics of being diffuse, achy and poorly localized. Think about the last time you had a stomach ache. Where was it? Sort of all over some part of your abdomen or most of your abdomen. You had no idea where this pain was originating from. The pain of the deep pain system often radiates at a distance away from the site of origin. Deep pain is difficult to describe.

All patients have difficulty describing deep pain. Why? When you are growing up and learning your colors, if you call something blue, which is actually red, you will immediately be corrected. You and I can look at a shirt which is not a primary color and decide to call the color of the shirt, "Colorado blue." I can call you from the other side of the world and tell you that I have seen a couch which is Colorado blue and you will know exactly what color it is. Why? We have both experienced the color, Colorado blue, together and can communicate to each other a word or phrase which names that color. I ignore for the moment people with color blindness. I also ignore for the moment the philosophical concerns about what we truly can know and what we can never be sure we know, well discussed by Rene Descartes and other philosophers.

There is never a time when two people have exactly the same pain or discomfort at the same time and know they are each having the same pain or discomfort at the same time. For this reason, our vocabulary for describing symptoms is limited, ambiguous and poorly defined. People have difficulty coming up with words which precisely describe their symptoms. Our language describing symptoms is vague and imprecise. There is never a time when I may use a word to describe a painful sensation when you or I can know if we are using that word in the same way.

Some of the symptom words commonly used to describe discomfort include: pain, discomfort, ache, nausea, numbness, tingling, headache, don't feel well, upset stomach, excruciating pain, soreness, throbbing, lightheaded, under the weather, cramping, burning, shooting, stabbing, unbearable pain, etc. Even though you may think that we all use these words alike, you have no way of knowing if this is true. In fact, it is certain that people use these words differently.

Back to taking our shoulder pain patient's history. After the patient responds with a description of the location of the pain or discomfort, you ask additional questions. You try to avoid suggesting answers. Follow up questions may include: Did you injure yourself? Does the pain stay in one place or does it travel? If so, where does it travel to? Have you ever had this problem before? Is the pain constant or does it come and go? If the pain is not constant, how does it vary? How often do you feel the pain? Is there any activity, movement or position, which makes the pain better or worse? Does anything trigger the pain? Does the pain limit your activity? Which activities aggravate your pain? Do you take any medicine for the pain? Does the pain medicine help? Does the pain prevent you from engaging in certain activities? Does the pain interfere with your sleep?

Depending on where the history taking has travelled, it is often useful to ask "Does anything else bother you?" or "Is there anything else you would like to discuss today?" As a hand surgeon I always ask about the presence or absence of numbness, tingling, pins and needles or "funny feelings." If I get a yes answer, I follow up with additional questions regarding the location, severity and characteristics of those additional symptoms. Carpal tunnel syndrome and cubital tunnel syndrome occur commonly. Asking after carpal tunnel syndrome symptoms and cubital tunnel syndrome symptoms including numbness, tingling, frequent dropping of objects and difficulty opening tight jar lids will pick up cases of both carpal tunnel syndrome and cubital tunnel syndrome.

I am not a fan of the one to ten number scale for describing the intensity of pain. It seems to me that, if the question of grading the pain on a number scale arises when I am seeing a new patient in my office, then the patient's self described number is usually five or greater. It seems that most patients feel that the pain should be labelled in the top half of possible pain to warrant an office visit with an orthopedic surgeon. I have seen numerous patients sitting in front of me on an examining table smiling, comfortable and clearly at ease, who tell me their pain is a nine or ten. Ten is supposed to be the worst possible pain you could ever have. Most people never experience a pain level of ten in their lifetime.

If a patient gives me a number, for example seven, and I ask the patient to describe for me their verbal definition of a pain level seven, I usually get a blank look in response. I get the same response if I ask a patient to explain the difference between a six and a seven on the pain scale. Try asking some of your patients the two questions above for yourself to see what kinds of responses you get.

In evaluating the severity of a patient's pain, I find that asking whether the patient takes medicine for the pain, if so, which medicine, does the medicine help the pain, how much does the medicine help the pain is more informative. Also, asking if the pain interferes with activities and how the pain interferes with activities are more helpful. Similarly asking if the pain interferes with sleep helps ascertain the level of severity. Asking the patient to draw a graph of the severity of pain with time may be useful, particularly in cases of chronic pain.

Back to the patient who complained of pain in shoulder. If the patient points to the neck then the pain is probably coming from the neck. If the patient points to the horizontal part between the neck and the point of the shoulder, you should consider the neck as the most likely cause. Neck pathology often presents with pain in the horizontal area between the neck and the point of the shoulder.

*Case Study:*

*Shortly after I entered the United States army as an orthopedic surgeon, a patient came in to the orthopedic clinic complaining of intermittent pain in the area between the neck and the point of the shoulder. He was an MP. That is, military police. One of his tasks was working at the entrance to the army base, waving cars in and out all day long. My patient complained of pain and a painful crunching sensation when waving the cars in and out of the base. Once again, the question: real or not real? Genuine or just trying to get out of work?*

*In fact, his initial complaint was accompanied with a dramatic demonstration that his shoulder "crunched" when he circumducted his shoulder before I even started my physical examination. The dramatic demonstration of his shoulder crunching was really part of this patient's self described medical history. I could hear the crunching noise across the room where I was sitting. I had never seen anything like this before. On examination there was distinct crunching crepitus at the upper medial corner of the scapula with circumduction of the shoulder joint.*

*An uncommon cause of pain in this area is snapping scapula syndrome. Occasionally the upper medial corner of the scapula curves sufficiently far anterior that the upper medial corner of the scapula impinges on the underlying ribs during active circumduction. I never saw a case in my training with this complaint or diagnosis. This diagnosis was never discussed in my training. I did not know that this syndrome existed when I walked into the examining room to evaluate this patient. No internet then to ease the search for information. I found a brief paragraph describing this in one of my textbooks.*

*My patient's symptoms were sufficiently severe and long standing to warrant surgery. I operated and removed the upper medial corner of the scapula. The patient had complete relief of pain. I ordered him to remain on light duty for three months after the surgery. He appeared in my office six weeks after the surgery begging to be allowed to return to full duty.*

*During the course of my career I have seen twenty or more cases of snapping scapula syndrome because I have been looking for it. I look for it in every shoulder exam I perform. For most patients the discomfort is minor and the crepitus is minor. They do not require surgical intervention or other treatment. For five other patients the discomfort was sufficiently severe that I operated similar to the case above with good results.*

*While in practice, I occasionally discussed this case with other orthopedic surgeons. No other orthopedic surgeon I talked to had seen any cases of snapping scapula syndrome. Why? They did not know of the existence of this syndrome. Thus, they did not know to look for this syndrome. Examining for snapping scapula syndrome was not part of their shoulder examination protocol.*

*Why mention this uncommon syndrome?*

*Thinking generally, if you do not know that a specific problem exists, you will not look for it. If you do not know that a specific problem exists, you will be unlikely to recognize it. I was fortunate that my first patient presented with a clear and precise history and a clear and precise demonstration of crepitus, I could hear across the room, without my needing to ask. Following my experience with this patient, I added the question, "Do you have any snapping or crunching when you move your shoulder?" to my routine shoulder history.*

Let's look at some patients who came to an orthopedic office complaining of lateral pain in the mid to lower back. All were seen by an internist first. All were referred to the orthopedic surgeon by an internist.

*Case Study:*

*A 38 year old woman is referred to my office for back pain. I ask the patient to point to where the pain hurts the most. As stated before, this is an important question which always provides useful information. The patient points to her right flank. The pain is far lateral, sort of posterior lateral lower thorax. This is an unusual location for "orthopedic" pain.*

*Here again is where the medical history and physical examination intermingle, intertwine, intersect. Due to the location of the pain my differential diagnosis starts out with concern for upper urinary tract problems such as a kidney stone, urinary tract infection or other ureteral blockage. My differential diagnosis also includes intra abdominal problems more likely involving the right upper quadrant of the abdomen. Percussion of the costo-vertebral angle is pain free. This does not rule out a blocked ureter but makes it a little less likely.*

*I continue my physical examination. Pain that far lateral in the lower thoracic area demands a careful examination of the abdomen. I repeat. Pain that far lateral in the lower thoracic area demands a careful examination of the abdomen. I repeat. Pain that far lateral in the lower thoracic area demands a careful examination of the abdomen.*

*There is some mild to moderate right upper quadrant tenderness to deep palpation. This tenderness increases somewhat with deep inspiration by the patient while I am palpating deeply in the right upper quadrant. I, the orthopedic surgeon, am now concerned that there is an abdominal cause to the right flank pain. Number one on my differential diagnosis is cholelithiasis. I am aware that there are a multitude of other possible causes of this clinical presentation. I, the orthopedic surgeon, order an abdominal sonogram. This was before the days of MRIs. The abdominal sonogram shows marked lymphadenopathy within the abdomen with a final diagnosis of lymphoma.*

This case study demonstrates the value of asking the patient where the pain hurts the most and then thoughtfully following up when the pain is in a non-standard location for your specialty. This case study demonstrates the importance of looking for diagnoses outside of your area of expertise. This case study also emphasizes that there are complaints of back pain that demand a physical examination of the abdomen.

*Case Study:*

*A patient is referred by an internist to one of my partners with a complaint of back pain. On close questioning the pain is far lateral, posterior lateral mid-thorax. This is not a common location for orthopedic pain. Mirabile dictu! My partner, an orthopedic surgeon, auscultates the lungs. My partner listens carefully to the lungs and hears a rub. He is concerned that something is irritating the outer surface of the lung where it moves against the pleura. He recommends a lung scan looking for possible pulmonary embolism. The internist initially resists ordering a lung scan. Lung scan, when obtained, shows a pulmonary embolism. Missing this diagnosis and not treating the patient with blood thinners would significantly increase the risk of this patient dying from another pulmonary embolism.*

Another case study which demonstrates the value of asking the patient where the pain hurts the most and then thoughtfully following up when the pain is in a location which suggests a problem outside of your specialty. This case study also highlights the need for you to be comfortable with the physical examination of areas outside of your specialty. This case study also highlights the importance of listening carefully when you are auscultating the chest. Rubs are soft and easy to miss.

*Case Study:*

*A patient is referred to me by a pulmonologist for evaluation of lateral chest pain of six weeks duration. Careful work up including several chest x-rays has been negative. The location of the pain is posterior and lateral lower thorax. I auscultate the chest. Normal. I obtain additional x-rays of the chest and ribs. Normal. What to do? The pain is not really "orthopedic" pain. The pulmonologist has referred the patient to me in desperation since he has been unable to diagnose the cause of the pain. I believe this patient's complaint is real. What to do? The patient seems "real." I believe his complaints of pain despite the normal work up so far. I order a CT scan of the chest. The CT scan shows a small cancer in the sulcus which has seeded the pleura. This is the cause of the pain.*

*The pulmonologist and I take all of our regular x-rays to a radiologist. We now know where the small cancer is located but we still cannot see it on the x-rays. The radiologist looks and tells us that even knowing where the cancer is, he is unable to detect it on the routine x-rays.*

If there is a lesson to be learned from this case study, the lesson is to listen to the patient when taking a history and decide when further tests are necessary. With a normal physical exam and normal x-rays, it would have been easy to brush off this patient. It would have been easy to state that further work up was unnecessary. Yet, taking a good history, listening to this patient and believing this patient's complaint allowed for me to make this diagnosis.

Other questions which are pertinent to all parts of the body include: What kind of work do you do? What do you actually do at work? What do you actually do at play? Have you recently engaged in any new or unaccustomed activity? If the patient's complaint involves the neck, back, shoulder, arm, hand, neck, back, hips, knees or feet: How do you use your arm and shoulder at work? How do you use your arm, shoulder and neck for other activities? How do you use your body at work and play? What position do you sleep in at night? If there is a skin rash, questions should include: Are you wearing new clothes, taking a new medicine, have you eaten new foods, etc.

*Case Study:*
*A woman was seen by a gynecologist for recurrent vulva vaginal candidiasis. She was having far more recurrences than normal. The gynecologist recognizes that this is a clear statistical outlier. Again, my use of the term statistical outlier. Finally, after multiple recurrences and thoughtful questioning by her gynecologist, the "cause" was discovered. This patient worked as a housekeeper in a*

*hotel. She spent much of her time washing and cleaning certain places which required her to use a lot of water. As a result, her clothes were constantly wet in front of her waist and perineal area. The persistent dampness of the front of her clothes led to an unusually moist environment around her perineum which allowed for the frequent candidiasis overgrowths. Arranging for a waterproof apron stopped the recurrences.*

If you don't recognize that a patient is presenting as a statistical outlier, if you don't recognize that there is a mystery, if you don't react to the knowledge that there is a mystery, if you don't follow up with detailed and thorough history taking you will not solve the mystery and successfully treat the patient.

*Case Study:*
*A woman came into my office complaining of chronic neck pain. History and work up were unremarkable. I finally asked her how she used her neck at work. She was a typist. She typed from handwritten documents converting the handwriting to typed copy. She placed the handwritten copy to her far right, so that as she was sitting all day her neck was fully rotated to the right. Why this positioning? Don't ask. I don't know. Once I obtained this information, I counseled her to move the handwritten documents forward so that they were just slightly to the right of her typewriter. Her pain went away. This was before the days of ubiquitous computers.*

*If I don't ask the question about how she is using or should I say abusing her neck, I won't figure out why her neck is hurting. Following extensive physical therapy and MRIs her neck will still hurt if I don't figure this out. An accurate, thorough history is necessary to make this diagnosis, i.e. find the cause of the neck pain. Multiple tests will not provide the answer.*

Here are more case studies emphasizing the importance of finding out how patients are using and abusing their bodies.

*Case Study:*

*A man in his 40s comes into my office complaining of chronic neck pain interfering with his work. X-rays and an MRI show degenerative changes consistent with age. Detailed history regarding how he uses his body. He works as a police photographer and often has to carry fifty pounds of photographic equipment half a mile to a crime scene in the woods. He is having difficulty doing this because of his neck pain. I encourage my patient to buy or make a large wheeled cart he can use to carry his equipment. He resists. The police macho thing, of course. After six months he comes in to see me. He has obtained a cart so that he no longer has to carry his equipment. His pain lessens. His pain is now sufficiently mild that he does not require further treatment. The fancy scan, that is the MRI findings, did not explain this patient's complaints. Successful evaluation and treatment required thoughtful questioning regarding his activities.*

*Case Study:*

*A 32 year old man came to my office complaining of diffuse aching in his right forearm. Physical examination in detail was negative. X-rays were negative. Then I took a "how do you use your arm at work and play" history. He replied that he was a graphic artist and used a "normal" computer mouse more than five hours a day. In order to use a "normal" computer mouse, one has to dorsiflex the wrist joint constantly. This means that the dorsal forearm muscles are in constant tension. Meanwhile, the shoulder muscles are constantly moving the mouse about and are in constant tension. The chronic tension of the dorsal forearm muscles and the chronic tension of the shoulder muscles causes chronic pain in some computer users.*

*The solution? I counseled the patient to obtain a computer mouse in which you rest your hand on the ulnar side of the hand and utilize your thumb on a ball to move the cursor around and your index and middle finger to click. Chronic forearm pain from "normal" computer mouse use is a common problem. I counseled patients to change their "mice" to another type of mouse more than one hundred times in my career. Many of these patients were graphic artists or performed similar work five or more hours a day on their computer.*

Any patient with a complaint of arm pain, for which the work up is unrevealing, should be questioned carefully regarding computer mouse use. Again, my refrain, scans won't show everything. Sometimes, careful history taking is key.

*Case Study:*

*A forty five year old woman came into my office complaining of bilateral hip pain. The pain was lateral to both hips. Physical examination showed tenderness over both greater trochanters. There was no pain on motion of the hip joint. X-rays were negative. She appeared to have bilateral greater trochanteric bursitis. Greater trochanteric bursitis is common. A presentation of unilateral greater trochanteric bursitis is common. A presentation of bilateral greater trochanteric bursitis is uncommon. That is, this presentation of bilateral greater trochanteric bursitis of the hip was a statistical outlier. Recognizing that the presentation of bilateral greater trochanteric bursitis was uncommon, that is, a statistical outlier. I took a detailed history, a "how are you using your body" history.*

*I inquired how she was using her hips and legs. She told me that she was walking for exercise. I asked how she was walking. She demonstrated an exaggerated method of walking. She took the longest possible stride that she was able to do. This involved externally rotating the back leg fully. She then reached as far forward with the swinging leg as possible. Then after planting the front leg, she swung the back leg around and as far forward as she was able to do, maximally externally rotating the now planted leg. This resulted in maximum external rotation of the front leg which became the back leg. Thus, with each stride, each hip was rotating maximally through internal and external rotation.*

*Her bursitis improved with cortisone shots. More importantly, my treatment involved counseling her to change her method of walking. The bursitis did not recur. If I don't figure out how she is using or abusing her body I will not permanently solve her problem.*

*Case Study:*

*A 37 year old woman comes in complaining of right hip pain. She is tender over the right greater trochanteric bursa. She clearly has right greater trochanteric bursitis. This is her third flare up. Hmm. Why is she having recurrent right hip bursitis? I ask questions regarding what are you doing a work and play. She is a runner. Now, I follow up with, "Where do you run?" She answers that she runs on the road. I follow up with, "Which side of the road do you run on?" She replies that she runs on the side facing traffic because it is safer.*

*Roads are not flat. They are subtly dome shaped to allow easy run off of rain. This means that all of her running is occurring on a subtly sloped surface with the right foot landing on a slightly higher surface than the left. This requires extra abduction of the right hip with each foot fall. This extra stress on the right hip is the reason that the right greater trochanteric bursitis is recurring. What was my treatment? I advise switching to running on a track, alternate sides of the street or if the street is deserted, running down the center of the street. The greater trochanteric bursitis does not recur.*

*Case Study:*

*A twelve year old boy comes into my office complaining of shoulder pain. He tells me he is a pitcher on a little league team. He spontaneously tells me his coach is careful to limit the number of times he pitches in a week. So, how should my history taking proceed? This is a true story. What was my first question after the patient finished talking? "How many teams do you pitch for?" The patient's answer: "Three."*

*With my first question I obtain the answer to why his shoulder is hurting. Each of the three coaches for each of the three baseball teams was careful to limit this boy to less than one hundred pitches a week. The cause: obvious overuse, i.e. abuse, of the shoulder. But, you have to know what questions to ask in order to find out. You have to be sufficiently knowledgeable regarding little league pitcher shoulder pain to ask the right questions. Failure to elicit the information that he is pitching for three teams will result in a failure of any treatment you provide.*

*Case Study:*
*Similarly, a fifteen year old boy comes to my office complaining of shoulder pain. He too is a pitcher. He only pitches for one team, his high school baseball team. His coach carefully counts pitches during each game and is careful to limit him to less than one hundred pitches per week. Hmmm. Is further questioning necessary? If so, what further questioning is necessary? I question further. After more questions, I elicit this information. My patient is also pitching for all of the batting practice for his team and those pitches are not being counted. The diagnosis: overuse of the shoulder. The diagnosis: abuse of the shoulder. The treatment, "Count all of your pitches!" and "Stop pitching too many pitches a week."*

*If I don't ask the right questions, if I don't push to obtain the important information, I will not figure out the "diagnosis" and will not solve the problem. My treatment will not be successful if I do not elicit the necessary information in my history.*

*Case Study:*
*A college freshman comes into my office complaining of pain on the lateral aspect of her right foot. Exam is normal except for mild tenderness on the lateral aspect of the fifth metatarsal. X-rays are normal. I ask questions about how she is using her foot. Finally. I obtain this information. She spends hours every day sitting cross legged on a hard floor chatting with her friends. Her right foot is underneath her legs and presses against the hard floor. You ask why she has not figured this out. I don't know. Once I elicit this history, I am able to treat her by telling her to stop sitting that way on a hard floor. If I don't ask the right questions, if I don't ask how she is using her body, if I don't figure this out her pain will continue. If I don't figure this out my treatment will not be successful.*

*Case Study:*

*I perform an operation for Dupuytren's contracture on a man's hand. I use a technique which leaves a transverse open wound in the distal palm, the McCash technique. These wounds all heal by themselves in about three weeks. That is, they all heal by themselves in about three weeks, except when they don't.*

*One time, I am confronted with a patient three weeks after his surgery with minimal evidence of healing of his hand wound. By this point in my career I have had extensive experience following the healing of the open wounds in patients after the McCash technique surgery. At three weeks after surgery, this patient's wound looks three days old. My antennae are quivering. Something is not right. I recognize that my patient's poor wound healing is a statistical outlier. I am intrigued. I ask many questions.*

*I finally stumble into questioning regarding diet and supplement intake. The patient is a strict vegetarian who eats predominantly salad and pasta. A detailed dietary history discloses minimal protein intake. My patient also takes a multitude of supplements including many different vitamin supplements. He describes a three foot long shelf of supplements. He takes one of each every day. I determine that he likely has a combination of protein intake insufficiency and hypervitaminosis. I counsel him to eat at least a palm size amount of meat every day and to stop all of his supplements. He follows my "treatment." His wound heals quickly.*

*If I don't recognize that this is a situation of unusually poor wound healing, if I don't recognize the fact that this patient's wound healing is a statistical outlier, if I don't actively respond to this recognition, I will not take a history sufficiently detailed to allow me to sort out the cause of the poor wound healing.*

*Case Study:*

*One of my partners admits a young man in his early twenties to the hospital. The patient has a two inch soft tissue open wound on his leg which does not go down to muscle. The wound is a month old and is not healing. A plastic surgery consult has been requested by my partner. I come in to see this patient on rounds the next day.*

*My antennae are quivering. I am intrigued. Why is this patient's wound not healing? A young healthy person should heal a wound like this quickly and effortlessly. I detect, I "observe" that this patient's poor wound healing is a statistical outlier.*

*I question him about diet and supplement intake. Initially, he answers that he eats a normal diet and takes no supplements. I tell him that I do not understand why he is not healing this wound. I tell him that I am concerned that if he is not healing this wound, then he will not heal his wound after plastic surgery. Then, as I am walking out of the room, the patient "confesses." He calls out, "Doc! Come back. I haven't eaten anything but Doritos for three months." This is a true story! Seriously. This is a true story! I make the diagnosis of protein and vitamin deficiency. I counsel him to eat a balanced diet including at least a palm size amount of meat each day and to take one multivitamin a day. I discharge him from the hospital. The patient follows my instructions and the wound heals quickly.*

*Case Study:*
*I see a patient with a "routine" fractured patella. One half of the patella is shattered into many fragments. The standard surgical treatment involves excision of the bone fragments and reconstruction of the extensor tendon mechanism with sutures anchored to the bone. A few weeks after surgery my repair dehisces and comes apart. My patient is unable to actively straighten his leg against gravity. This is an operation I have done frequently without ever having a single complication. Suddenly, I have a patient with this complication. I ask myself, "Why?" I ask myself why has this patient had this complication. I consider this occurrence of dehiscence of my surgical repair to be a statistical outlier for my personal orthopedic surgery experience.*

*I take a detailed history. The two cases of improper diet and/or vitamin and supplement intake causing wound healing complications I described previously are not the only ones I have seen. I sense that this patient may be another. I immediately take a dietary and supplement intake history. My patient is a salad and pasta eater. He reports essentially no protein intake and little vitamin intake. I diagnose combined protein deficiency and vitamin deficiency. Note the existence of additional diagnoses in this patient who initially presented with a "straight-forward" patellar fracture.*

*I counsel my patient to eat a palm size amount of meat per day as medicine and to take one multivitamin a day. After a week I operate and repair the dehiscence. This time the surgical repair heals without complication.*

*If I don't recognize the fact that the complication is unusual, if I don't recognize the fact that the complication is a statistical outlier, I won't take a detailed history regarding diet and vitamin intake, I will not find a solution to this problem. Not only that but the patient would probably fail to heal after a second operation.*

Be aware. There are many salad and pasta eaters out there. They do not heal well after injuries and surgery, probably due to protein deficiency. Some have vitamin deficiency. Some have hypervitaminosis from taking too many vitamins and supplements. Find these patients before you operate on them. This case occurred before I became aware that poor dietary, vitamin and supplement intake are more common problems than generally realized.

At times questions such as, "Where do you live?" "Where have you lived?" and "Where have you travelled to?" are important.

*Case Study:*
*Me. My chest x-ray shows multiple small densities scattered throughout my lung fields. Question: "Where have you lived?" Answer: "I grew up in Cincinnati which is in the Ohio River Valley." The fungus, histoplasmosis, is prevalent*

*in the Ohio and Mississippi River valleys. I had a bad case of "pneumonia" as a child and recall being in bed for three weeks. In medical school we planted PPDs on our forearms to test for TB. We used histoplasmosis as the "control." Bad idea! My PPD was negative, no reaction. My histoplasmosis "control" had a severe reaction and I almost had necrosis of tissue. The history of "where I lived" explains my chest x-ray findings and my histoplasmosis skin test findings.*

Certain construction workers may be more at risk for asbestosis. Coal miners are more at risk for black lung disease. In the early 20th century the "Radium Girls" were women who painted watch faces with paint containing radium. They were instructed to use their lips to narrow the points of the brushes. Many later suffered and died with anemia, bone fractures and necrosis of the jaw.

I find it curious that my experience with asking patients about exposure to possible tick borne diseases was rarely useful. Of the patients I saw with swollen wrists, knees or ankles who had positive Lyme tests, I only recall one who reported walking in the woods. None reported the classic bullseye rash. I obviously was seeing a subset of Lyme disease patients whose first symptoms were swollen joints. I still asked after activities risky for tick bites because I thought I should, but I was aware that I was probably wasting time. If I was far enough along in my evaluation that I was thinking of a possible tick borne disease, then I was going to order the tests anyway. Patients with hanta virus infections often report exposure to situations involving dried rat feces.

Observing. Observing. Always observing. Recognizing when something is not standard. Recognizing when something is a statistical outlier. Then, acting on those observations and recognitions. These are the steps, the actions, the behaviors necessary for the excellent practice of medicine.

In this coming age of increasingly complex scans, diagnostic tests and the use of artificial intelligence, of what use is the patient history? The many vignettes above demonstrate that many problems will only be solved by careful observation by the medical provider, by thoughtful history taking and by thorough physical examinations. With time, artificial intelligence will assist in history taking and in a far distant future may take over history taking completely. For the present, careful observation, careful history taking and careful physical examinations are still crucial to the practice of excellent medicine and surgery.

The critical problem in history taking is often figuring out what question or questions to ask. In the case of the post operative Dupuytren's contracture patient mentioned before, I recognized that something was amiss because the wound was not healing properly. I recall asking a great many questions trying to find the cause of the failure to heal properly. I finally stumbled onto the improper diet and excess vitamin intake cause. Since then I have found dietary and supplement intake as a cause of poor wound healing and poor fracture healing in perhaps twenty patients. Taking a dietary and supplement intake history has become a frequent occurrence in my practice. This possibility was never discussed or covered in my training. I had to figure it out for myself.

I think that a careful dietary intake and vitamin and supplement intake history should be part of every yearly checkup. I think that a careful dietary intake and vitamin and supplement intake history should be part of every preoperative evaluation. I think that a careful dietary intake and vitamin and supplement intake history should be part of the evaluation of any surgical complication. I believe that poor diet and improper vitamin and supplement intake are a greater cause of health issues and postoperative complications than is generally recognized. I also believe that poor diet and poor vitamin intake are contributing causes in the deterioration of elderly patients with early cognitive decline who stop eating a proper diet.

Here is one last vignette in which finding the correct question to ask was difficult.

*Case Study:*

*This case probably dates to the 1930s. My father was a pediatrician in Cincinnati and told me this story from his practice. He saw a child with scurvy. Scurvy is lack of Vitamin C which is present in orange juice. My father asked the child's mother if she was giving her child orange juice. She replied that she was. My father could not understand how his patient continued to suffer from scurvy when her mother was giving her orange juice.*

*I believe it took my father some time, a few office visits and many questions before he finally asked the child's mother what she was doing with the orange juice when she gave it to her child. The patient's mother replied that she was boiling the orange juice to sterilize it. This sounds crazy to you, I know. But, the family was living on a farm and they boiled the milk they got from their cows. That is called pasteurization. It is not that farfetched to understand that they were boiling the orange juice to sterilize it as well. Boiling destroys Vitamin C. Only by figuring out what question or questions to ask will you sort out such conundrums. Diagnostic problems like this will not be solved with sophisticated scans and lab tests.*

Why have I presented these many vignettes demonstrating the difficulty of making unusual diagnoses. During the course of a long career you may see tens of thousands of patients. If you are not careful, if you are not thoughtful and if you are not curious about each and every patient, even the apparently plain and mundane patients, particularly the plain and mundane patients, you will miss diagnoses, you will be an average medical provider, you will be an ordinary medical provider rather than an outstanding one. Attitude and care count.

I recognize that I am being preachy. I recognize that practicing excellent medicine is hard. I am hectoring you because I have seen and personally encountered too much "ordinary" medicine in my life. I also present these many vignettes to help you understand exactly how wild, wacky and wonderful the clinical practice of medicine can be. Figuring out one of these unusual diagnoses is exhilarating. It makes practicing medicine fun.

A patient's use of certain words may be ambiguous. A doctor's use of certain words may be ambiguous. The same word may be used and understood differently by different people. For example, some people use the word "pain" only to describe a symptom which is severe. Others may use the word "pain" to describe symptoms which are mild. Probably 95% of patients coming to see a general orthopedic surgeon complain of pain or discomfort somewhere in their body. The others complain of a painless bump or inability to move a part of their body.

I recall early in my career asking patients if they were having any pain and being told "No." Confused, I then asked, "Well then, why are you here?" I was then told that the patient was having discomfort. Having learned that the word "pain" is used differently by people, I now follow up a "No" answer to my "Are you having any pain?" with the question "Are you having any discomfort?" The patients who say "No" to the pain question often immediately answer 'Yes" to the "Are you having any discomfort?" question. The history taking then continues. You can bypass this possible ambiguity by asking, "Are you having any pain or discomfort?" This was the question I drifted to with time and experience.

Another source of ambiguity in talking with patients is the use of the phrase, "I will see you next Wednesday." Assume today is Monday. There is a sizable group of people who will say that "next Wednesday" is two days away. An equally sizable group of people will say that "next Wednesday" is nine days away. When asked, the first group will say that the Wednesday in two days is the "next" Wednesday. When asked, the second group will say that the Wednesday in two days is "this" Wednesday and the Wednesday in nine days is, therefore, the "next" Wednesday. Recognizing this potential ambiguity will allow you to communicate with patients clearly.

We all have difficulty describing symptoms to each other. If fact, we have difficulty describing any sensations to each other. When trying to describe colors, we find the description easier if we can refer to another well known color. For example, "robin's egg blue." Trying to describe an unusual "off" color to someone who has not seen that color is difficult. A person hearing that attempted description who has not seen the "off" color who is then asked to create that color by mixing paints will not be able to recreate that color.

Similarly, trying to describe the sound of a train or a helicopter to someone who has never heard those sounds is near impossible if the describer is prevented from recreating the sound. Try describing the taste of a brownie hot fudge sundae (with real hot fudge, not some sweet chocolate syrup imitation) (particularly as served on Cape Cod) to someone who has never tasted hot fudge, ice cream, or brownies. Can't do it. You can tell I am partial to brownie hot fudge sundaes and Cape Cod. Note, I left the whipped cream out of the description to avoid diluting the chocolate taste with the whipped cream. Sorry, I think I got distracted. Don't forget to ask for extra hot fudge. If you don't ask for extra hot fudge, you will run out of hot fudge while you still have ice cream and brownie left.

Everyone has experienced touch. Thus, you can describe a new touch sensation to someone else by comparing that touch sensation to a similar touch sensation you both have experienced.

There is never a time when two people have exactly the same ache, cramp, pain, numbness, tingling or other internal sensation and know this is happening simultaneously. Thus, there is never a time when two people can invent or agree on the use of a word or words to describe internal sensations and know that they are using a descriptive sensation word to name the same sensation. As a result, our vocabulary for describing internal sensations or symptoms is vague, ambiguous and limited. Many patients have trouble coming up with symptom descriptive words. Patients for whom English is a second language will have even greater difficulty trying to describe their symptoms in English or via a translator.

If a patient is having difficulty describing symptoms and internal sensations, the issue may not be the patient's intelligence, vocabulary or use of English, the issue may simply be the fact that the symptoms are really hard to describe.

*Case Study:*
*Me. In my late 40s I fell while skiing and injured my left shoulder. For the first hour or two the pain in my left shoulder was what I describe as "typical" musculoskeletal injury pain. I have hurt myself before. Not a great description. Even though I am an orthopedic surgeon, that is the best I can do. My pain was localized to the left shoulder area and was increased with motion of my shoulder.*

*Within an hour or two the character of the pain changed. It became more intense and radiated into my left upper arm. The character of the pain also changed. This later pain was "weird." The first pain was a pain my brain could "understand." The later pain was a pain my brain could "not understand." Those are the only words I can use to describe the new pain. The new pain was "weird", "unpleasant" and "annoying." Again, a remarkably limited description.*

*Five days later, I developed a linear vesicular rash on my anterior left shoulder and upper arm making the diagnosis of shingles and confirming that my pain was coming from the onset of post herpetic neuropathy. I am trained in questioning patients about their pain, yet I am "descriptionless" when trying to describe the unpleasant sensations I had at that time.*

*Case Study:*
*Me. Me again. In my early 70s I developed "weird" and "unpleasant" sensations in my brain which were diagnosed as vestibular migraines by several physicians, although I never had spinning sensations. I did have a few episodes of cataclysmic vomiting and difficulty holding my head upright. Again, my use of the words "weird" and "unpleasant" but no actual, useful description. My symptoms went away after about six months and have not returned. Again, my absolute inability to describe in any meaningful way, the symptoms I was feeling. I have had personal experience with unpleasant sensations in my body*

*for which I am starkly and profoundly unable to provide a description. Our language does not contain such descriptive words.*

If I, a trained orthopedic and hand surgeon, am unable to describe my "discomfort" then why should I expect any of my patients to be able to do so. When questioning patients about pain, discomfort or other unpleasant sensations expect a lack of ability to describe their symptoms, such as I have documented above.

At times it is important and necessary to ask "awkward" questions, particularly about sexual exposure history.

*Case Study:*
*A federal judge (long since deceased) many, many years ago developed swelling of one of his wrist joints. He consulted a rheumatologist. Over the course of the following year, the judge consulted a total of three rheumatologists concerning his swollen, painful wrist. The three rheumatologists were excellent physicians by reputation. None were able to make a definitive diagnosis. None of their treatments were successful. Over the course of a year x-rays documented the progressive destruction of the wrist joint until there was no joint space at all.*

*Finally, the judge consulted a fourth rheumatologist. This rheumatologist as part of his history taking protocol took a sexual exposure history from this federal judge. I was told that the judge freely admitted frequenting prostitutes on a weekly basis. The diagnosis made by the fourth rheumatologist? Chronic untreated gonorrhea infection of the wrist joint. By the time the judge consulted the fourth rheumatologist the wrist joint was completely destroyed by the infection due to the delay in making the correct diagnosis.*

*The gonococcus bacteria requires a specific growth medium in order for a culture to successfully grow out the bacteria. Thus, previous cultures of fluid aspirated from the wrist joint were negative because gonococcus was not considered and the joint fluid sample was not cultured in the proper medium.*

*I saw this patient in consultation as a hand surgeon shortly after the diagnosis was made and following antibiotic therapy. I was consulted for the question of what treatment to recommend for the destroyed wrist joint. I recommended a wrist arthrodesis.*

*Due to the perceived awkwardness regarding taking a sexual exposure history from a federal judge, the diagnosis was missed by three otherwise excellent physicians. The omission of taking a sexual exposure history, the failure to take a sexual exposure history from this federal judge led to the failure to make the diagnosis. The first three rheumatologists failed to follow their history taking protocol by failing to ask about the sexual exposure history of a federal judge in evaluating a swollen wrist joint. Or. Perhaps taking a sexual exposure history was not part of their spontaneous, swollen wrist history taking protocol. Only the fourth rheumatologist got it right.*

I will discuss the issue of making and following protocols in history taking, physical examination performing and in treatment situations later. Making your own personal protocols as you go through your training and then following those protocols rigidly will make you a better medical provider. As you progress in your training you will need to decide the situations in which taking a sexual exposure history is necessary. A spontaneous swollen joint is certainly one of them.

The approach to medical history taking in any patient varies depending on the age of the patient. The approach to medical history taking also depends on the purpose of the interaction with the patient, i.e. yearly well checkup or evaluation of a specific complaint. The approach to medical history taking also varies depending on the part of the body or anatomic system which seems to be involved. Other issues which may influence how the history is taken may include possible psychiatric issues, questions of physical abuse and questions of sex trafficking to name a few.

Age is always a critical factor in evaluating a patient. Thus, complaints of persistent vomiting in a six week old baby raises the question of pyloric stenosis. Whereas persistent vomiting in a fifteen year old girl raises the question of early pregnancy as well as a multitude of gastrointestinal disorders.

Hip pain in an infant six to thirty six months old raises the question of septic arthritis of the hip. In a six year old the hip pain is more likely caused by Legg Calve Perthes disease or toxic synovitis of the hip. In a tall or obese fourteen year old slipped capital femoral epiphysis is a more likely cause of hip pain. In a 35 year old, bursitis. In a 55 year old degenerative arthritis of the hip. And so on. My point is that the moment you combine the age of the patient with the complaint, for example hip pain, the differential diagnosis in your mind changes completely.

If there is any question of abuse, eg. physical, mental or sex trafficking, it is important to isolate the patient and question that patient alone. If the patient's presentation suggests the need for sexual exposure history questions, you need to ask family members or parents to step outside, so that you can question the patient alone. This may be necessary for young teenagers.

# CHAPTER SIX:

# Taking the complete medical history

## The review of systems

Perhaps I should have placed this chapter at the beginning of my discussion on the taking of the medical history. I was more interested in presenting to you the challenge, the art, the science and the fun of medical history taking as well as discussing the philosophy, the psychology and the proper attitude of taking a medical history than I was interested in discussing the medical history from an organized, structured point of view. Here is an organized, structured discussion of the taking of the medical history.

A complete medical history includes the chief complaint, the history of present illness, the past medical history, review of systems, social history, family history, known imaging studies, known laboratory studies, impression and treatment plan. The history of present illness may include previous hospitalizations and surgeries related to the current problem. The past medical history includes more or less everything else including hospitalizations and surgeries for other reasons.

In my training, the complete medical history did not cover the vaccination status of the patient. We need to evolve and adapt to changes in our world. Vaccination status deserves, I believe, a separate category of its own in any complete medical history.

As stated earlier, in my training diet, vitamin and supplement intake history was ignored in taking a medical history. I think diet, vitamin and supplement intake history should also have a specific category of its own in any complete medical history.

In this book, I am not trying to cover everything you will see and do. That would require a constantly updated multi-volume textbook. My goal is to give you an introduction, an attitude, an approach, a philosophy to help guide you in learning the basics and the intricacies of the art and science of taking a medical history and performing a physical examination.

Taking a review of systems from a patient is a method of looking for symptoms which may be important but about which the patient is not concerned. No specific order of questioning is necessarily better than another. You will find that the printed forms or the computer program you use for electronic medical records may have its own order you are expected to follow.

As in all medical history taking it is important to use words the patient understands. For example:

Don't ask: "Have you had any dyspnea?"
Ask instead: "Have you had any difficulty breathing or shortness of breath?"

Don't ask: "Have you had any dysuria?"

Ask instead: "Do you have difficulty peeing, pain when peeing or difficulty getting your pee stream to start?

I am going to provide a list of review of system questions. This list is not meant to be complete. In most cases it may be too time consuming to ask everything I have listed. This list is meant to give you a start to learning the kinds of questions you will need to ask. Obviously, any yes answer to a review of systems question requires follow up questions.

Constitutional questions

Do you have any history of unexplained fevers, sweats, chills, weight loss, fatigue, malaise, lethargy?

Any past history of cancer?

Has your exercise tolerance unchanged?

Are you able to walk and run the way you used to?

Has there been any recent changes I should know about?

Has there been any change in the way you feel generally?

Has there been any change in your sleeping pattern?

Do you get out of breath walking upstairs or up a hill?

Do you get out of breath when you lie down?

For any yes answers you obviously switch to follow up questions.

When did something start?

How much does it bother you?

Is it there all of the time or does it come and go? Etc.

The nature and tenor of the questions varies with the patient's age. For an elderly patient, you should ask general questions such as:

Are you falling often?

Are you having trouble remembering things?

Are you forgetting to pay your bills?

For the young child, you may ask, "Where is your booboo?" or "Where is your tummy ache?"

Psychiatric, Psychologic

Do you feel more happy or more sad?

If unhappy, have you considered ending your life?

If so, have you considered how you might do that?

Do you feel unusually anxious or afraid?

Have you ever sought psychiatric care or hospitalization?

Mental-Cognitive ability

This will be covered in more detail in the neurologic examination section.

Ask the patient for his/her name, location, time, name of the current president.

Ask "Have you gotten lost while driving?

Are you forgetting to pay your bills?

Have you lost your car keys?

Are you having trouble remembering things?

Eyes

Are you having any trouble with your vision?

Can you see as well as you use to?

Are you having floaters or flashes of light in your eyes?

Are you having any headaches, double vision, eye pain or blind spots?

Ears, Nose and Throat

Are you having increased difficulty hearing someone talking in another room?

Do you have trouble with a stuffy nose?

Do you have frequent sore throats?

Have you had any recent changes in your voice?

Do you have sinus pain, ear pain, constant runny nose, frequent nose bleeds?

Do you have ringing in your ears, stuffy ears, mouth sores, pain with swallowing or difficulty swallowing?

Cardiovascular-Central

Have you had chest pain, difficulty breathing, shortness of breath, wheezing, coughing, fainting spells or irregular heart beat?

Do you have or have you ever had pneumonia, asthma, bronchitis?

Do you ever feel your heart racing or have an irregular pulse?

Do your feet and ankles swell?

Do you have or have you had episodes of palpitation, sudden loss of consciousness or feelings of faintness?

Do you have trouble walking upstairs or up a hill?

Do you get out of breath when you lie down?

Vascular-peripheral

Are you having trouble walking distance?

Can you run as far as you used to?

Is there a limit to how far you can walk or run without stopping?

Can you walk as far as you used to?

Do your fingers ever go white in color?

Do you get ulcers on your legs?

Respiratory

Do you have problems with coughing, wheezing, shortness of breath, sputum production or recent exposure to someone with cough or pulmonary illness?

Has there been any change in your exercise tolerance?

Are you having trouble walking distance?

Can you run as far as you used to?

Is there a limit to how far you can walk or run without stopping?

Do you get out of breath walking upstairs or up a hill?

Can you walk as far as you used to?

Are you bringing up a lot of sputum? If so, "What color is it."

Do you ever cough up blood?

Do you get out of breath when you lie down?

## Gastrointestinal

Do you have any problems with nausea, vomiting or diarrhea?

Do you ever have abdominal pain?

Have you lost weight recently without trying to?

Do you feel the need to have bowel movements at night that awaken you from sleep?

Do you have increased difficulty swallowing, increased frequency of bowel movements, urgency in getting to the toilet for bowel movements, altered consistency of your bowel movements, decreased appetite, bloating, or food intolerance?

Have you vomited blood, had bright red blood in your stools or had black tarry stools?

## Dermatology

Do you have any problems with rashes, history of inflammatory arthritis or any lesions which are getting larger, have an irregular shape or coloring or that you are worried about?

If the patient has a rash, "Have you ever been told you have arthritis?"

## Rheumatology-Allergy-Autoimmune

Have you ever been told that you have any kind of arthritis?

Do any of your joints have problems with swelling, redness, stiffness or limited motion?

Are you stiff in the morning when you awaken?

If so, "How long does the stiffness last?

Have you ever had choking, wheezing, difficulty breathing or air hunger after exposure to anything such as a bee sting, a specific food, an article of clothing or anything else?

Genito-Urinary

Do you have pain when you urinate?

Do you have difficulty initiating your urine flow?

Are you urinating more frequently than usual?

For men:

"Are you able to reach the back of the toilet bowl when you urinate?

Do you have difficulty holding your urine in until your reach a toilet?

Do you leak urine when you cough or sneeze?

Do you use contraception and protection when engaging in intercourse?

Do you have pain when you urinate?

For women:

When was your last menstrual period?

Are your periods regular or irregular?

Other than during your menses, do you have vaginal bleeding?

If so, how frequently do you need to change pads?

How many children have you had?

Were your children delivered vaginally or by cesarean section?

Do you use contraception and protection when engaging in intercourse?

Are you having increased vaginal discharge or pain or irritation around your vagina?

Do you have pain with intercourse?

Does your bladder push outwards when you cough or sneeze?

Musculoskeletal

Are you having or have you had neck pain or back pain?

Do you have any lumps, bumps or masses I should look at?

Do you have any joint swelling, stiffness, limited motion or grinding when you move your joints?

Are you able to walk or run as far as you used to?

Endocrine

Do you have difficulty with hot or cold environments?

Do you urinate frequently?

Have you had high blood pressure which has been difficult to treat?

There are many other endocrine related questions. A complete list is beyond the scope of this book.

Neurology

Have you ever had a seizure or stroke?

Do you feel that your arms or legs are weaker than they should be?

Are you having trouble with maintaining your balance?

Are you having difficulty walking or feeding yourself?

Do you have trouble walking?

Hematology-Oncology-Lymphatic

Any history of unusual bleeding, blue spots on your skin, easy bruising or family history of bleeding disorders? Note: This question should be asked before any surgery, elective or not.

Do you have increased frequency of urination?

Are you frequently thirsty?

For someone who is not a senior: Are you getting up at night to pee?

Are you sensitive to hot or cold temperatures?

Vaccination

When I was in practice taking a vaccination history was ignored. Today, I think a vaccination history is a necessary part of the medical history. If a patient has ignored or avoided vaccines, you know that part of your "treatment" needs to be counseling regarding the benefits of vaccinations. Thus, asking after vaccinations for Hepatitis A, B and C, childhood vaccinations, Covid, flu, pneumovax and shingles are important among others.

Family History

Your questioning should cover any family history of diagnoses which have familial tendencies including heart disease, cancers and known inherited disorders.

Social History

This covers life style and the use of mind altering substances. Why is this important? A chronic alcoholic has a serious risk of developing delirium tremens if admitted to a hospital and abruptly taken off alcohol intake. Similarly, a drug addict may go into withdrawal if admitted to a hospital and abruptly taken off drugs. A child being raised in commune environment may not be getting the needed vaccinations.

What kind of situation is an ill patient or patient being discharged from a hospital going home to?

Asking after foreign travel looks for exposure to diseases which are rare in the United States.

Dietary History, Vitamin and Supplement Intake

I am not sure where to put questions about diet and vitamin and supplement intake. I am personally giving diet and vitamin and supplement intake a section of their own. You will not find that in other lists of topics for a review of systems. I, personally, think this is sufficiently important to deserve a section of its own. That way it will not be overlooked.

Patients with strict, limited diets should be evaluated for possible deficiency syndromes. For patients who take supplements finding out what supplements they take and where they get the supplements from may be important. Finding out how much of which vitamins patients take is also important. At times, finding out where your patient is obtaining her medicine from may be important.

*Case Study:*

*I am evaluating a one armed patient in my office. He lost his other arm in a severe accident as a child. His remaining arm has severe carpal tunnel syndrome. His remaining hand has distinct thenar atrophy. His electromyographic studies show significant denervation of the median nerve innervated muscles with fasciculations. He needs carpal tunnel release surgery. We, both, are understandably nervous when considering operating on the only hand of a one handed patient. Still, it needs doing.*

*As I discuss surgery with my patient, I take a detailed social history. I ask, "Do you have anyone to help take care of you immediately after surgery?" He answers, "No." As part of his preoperative preparation, I arrange for his admission to a rehabilitation facility for a week and a half after surgery until his stitches are removed. He cannot care for himself alone with a bandaged hand after surgery. For this patient taking a careful social history was a necessary part of his preoperative evaluation.*

*Case Study:*

*I am taking a medical history in my first months of clinical training. My patient is a woman who is a chronic alcoholic. She has been sober for two years. I say in my naive eagerness, "Your husband must have been thrilled when you stopped drinking." She replies, "Oh, no. He lost a drinking partner." We rarely know much about the social environment our patients live in.*

*Case Study:*

*Told to me by a visiting nurse. Her patient was a man with severe disabling rheumatoid arthritis. His wife was taking care of his in home care including help with bathing and feeding. The patient owned the house and paid for the taxes and maintenance. Also, living in the same house was the wife's boyfriend. The husband paid for the shelter and food for the wife and boyfriend. The wife cared for the husband. Such was their mutual living arrangement. We rarely know much about the social environment our patients live in.*

68

*Case Study:*
*Told to me by the same visiting nurse. An elderly man had fallen in his home several times with resulting fractures. The house was filled with multiple small throw rugs which were serious fall hazards. The wife ignored the visiting nurse's entreaties to remove the small rugs. The elderly man continued to fall. We rarely know much about the social environment our patients live in.*

Issues with drug addiction, sexual abuse, violence, neglect etc. are often present and need to be considered when and where possible.

# CHAPTER SEVEN:
# The physical examination

Now, I move on to discussing the physical examination. Classically, we are taught that every general physical examination includes observation, auscultation, palpation and percussion. Auscultation is most useful in examining the heart, lungs and abdomen. Auscultation is also useful in listening for bruits especially in the carotid arteries and aorta. A continuous bruit may be heard over the thyroid in cases of hyperthyroidism.

Percussion is useful in examining the thoracic cavity for pleural effusions, in examining the abdominal cavity looking for hepatomegaly, splenomegaly and bladder distention. Percussion is not used often enough in postoperative and post trauma patients looking for possible urinary retention. Even females may suffer postoperative urinary retention, though much less commonly than males.

Percussion of the lower abdomen should be part of the physical examination every day in patients recovering from big surgeries, abdominal surgery, spine surgery and trauma. I have encountered missed bladder retention on a remarkably frequent basis during my entire career. For reasons I do not understand, surgeons, physicians and nurses seem to ignore the possibility of urinary retention following surgery or trauma and don't actively look for it.

When you are in the hospital please keep the possibility of postoperative or post trauma urinary retention in mind and actively look for it by percussing for a distended bladder. Ask yourself whether there is dullness to percussion from the pubis up to the umbilicus. If there is, the bladder is probably distended. Bladder scans are now easily available but you always have your two middle fingers available for percussion. You don't leave home without them.

Seriously, of all of the issues concerning inpatients that I discovered, which were missed by other medical providers, unrecognized urinary retention is far and away the most common.

*Case Study:*
*A family member was admitted to the hospital for spine surgery. The following morning when I came in to see her, I noted that she was voiding frequently with small amounts. This is a "classic" symptom of urinary retention. I percussed her bladder up to the umbilicus. When the spine surgeon came by on rounds and when a nurse came by, I asked both of them to perform a bladder scan to look for urinary retention. They knew I was a surgeon, yet they still ignored me. Finally, after eight more hours of urinary retention in my family member, I agitated and demanded a bladder scan which indeed showed urinary retention. Why the spine surgeon and the nurse were resistant to my earlier polite requests, I do not understand. Medical providers just seem to ignore the possibility of urinary retention in my experience.*

Other parts of the physical examination which are not part of the classic four may include provocative maneuvers such as the Adson's Test, Tinel's Sign, straight leg raising test, femoral stretch test, multiple tests for joint ligament instability, grind tests for pain, eg patella femoral joint, and thumb carpal metacarpal joint. These provocative tests will be covered as I discuss the physical examination of the various parts of the body. Cardiac stress tests and pulmonary function tests are simply more complicated and more sensitive provocative tests.

A complete physical examination may also include measurements such as the circumference of the thighs, calves, chest excursion and leg lengths. Measurement of the circumference of the thighs may be useful in evaluating rehabilitation following knee surgery, evaluating lymphedema and possible limb size discrepancy. Measurement of the calves and ankles may be useful in evaluating possible phlebitis, lymphedema, limb size discrepancy and recovery from congestive heart failure with peripheral edema of the legs and feet. Measurement of chest excursion in young males with spine or joint pain may be useful in picking up patients with ankylosing spondylitis. You measure the circumference of the chest from full expiration to full inspiration. A measured excursion of less than one inch demands evaluation for ankylosing spondylitis. Leg length measurements may be useful in evaluating questions of leg length discrepancy and pelvic tilt.

The details of any physical examination depend on the circumstances of the encounter between the medical provider and the patient. As I discuss the details of various physical examination situations, I make no attempt to be "complete." I am trying to be sufficiently thorough that I am able to give you a head start toward your approach to physical examination of the patient. If I have left out some part of the physical examination which you feel is important, I apologize. I know I can't please everyone.

For all physical examinations careful, thoughtful, heightened aware observation is key. For all physical examinations do not just go through the rote motions. For all physical examinations ask yourself at each step specific questions such as, "Do I hear a heart murmur?" "Do I hear a heart rub?" "Do I hear a pleural rub?" "Is the liver enlarged or tender?" and so on. For all physical examinations be observant, be thoughtful, be careful. Look for abnormalities.

**The physical examination of any patient should start with Observation, Observation, Observation.**

Physical Examination in an Emergency

In an emergency situation with an unconscious patient, checking the airway and checking for heart beat are the instant priorities. Urgently deciding whether CPR is necessary is the priority.

*Case Study:*
*I am just beginning to talk with a new patient in my office when she says, "I feel faint. I feel faint. I feel faint." I immediately lie her down on the floor and elevate her legs on a chair. I have been taught that you can't faint if you are lying down. She repeats, "I feel faint." Then her eyeballs click up and she becomes unconscious. I know that her airway is open because she has been talking normally. I palpate her radial pulse. She has a good normal pulse. She continues to breathe normally. Airway, breathing and heart function are normal for the moment. I do not understand why she has lapsed into unconsciousness. However, my emergent evaluation of (ABC) airway, breathing and cardiac function informs me that I can wait a few minutes before calling 911. After about a minute her eyelids flicker and she awakens. She tells me, "I must have had a seizure." This was a petit mal seizure. She had a known history of petit mal seizures which I had not yet gotten to in my medical history.*

*Case Study:*
*I am a general surgery intern. I answer my beeper and my senior resident informs me that a patient we are expecting has just arrived on ward D2. We know this patient has postoperative complications following surgery at another hospital and has renal failure. I run up to Ward D2. As I arrive two other physicians arrive at the bedside, the head of respiratory care and his fellow. We start to talk to the patient. We start our medical history. Less than five minutes pass. The patient suddenly becomes limp and unconscious. A few seconds and we determine that there is no heart beat and no spontaneous breathing. We initiate immediate CPR. This is or perhaps I should say was the immediate "limited" emergency physical examination. Unconscious. No heartbeat. No breathing.*

*Start immediate CPR. This CPR was successful although it took half an hour. More details of this case are given in "The Qi of the Scalpel."*

*The emergency physical examination concerns the questions: Is the heart beating? Is the patient breathing? If not, chest compression is begun immediately, then the airway is checked for obstruction, then breathing for the patient.*

The two cases above demonstrate the use of the immediate, emergency, "limited" physical examination evaluation.

In general, the age of the patient and the purpose of the examination, i.e. general checkup or complaint specific, determines the type and details of the physical examination.

Routine evaluation of newborn

The first part of the physical examination of a newborn baby is, of course, observation. You look at color. Initial cyanosis is normal. Persistent cyanosis may be a sign of a congenital heart defect and requires further evaluation. Does the baby have a good strong cry? For example, a high pitched cry, the cri du chat or cry of the cat, is a sign of a specific chromosomal abnormality. Does the baby have a normal flexed posture? Is the baby's size consistent with gestational age?

Some head bruising is normal. Fontanels should be soft. Sutures may overlap. There should be free, full motion of the neck. Swelling and/or crepitus and/or tenderness around a clavicle may indicate a clavicle fracture. Examine the palate for clefts. Examine the lingua frenulum of the tongue for shortening or abnormal attachment. If present, this may interfere with breast feeding. Breathing should be easy and not labored with a respiratory rate of 40-60 breaths per minute. Auscultate of the heart to listen for abnormal murmurs. Heart rate should be 120-160 beats per minute. Auscultate the abdomen. Bowels sounds should be normal. Genitalia should have normal size and structure. Examine the back for symmetry, skin lesions and spinal dysra-phisms. Arms and legs should have normal structure. Look for abnormalities such as club feet.

Utilize provocative maneuvers for assessing possible developmental hip dysplasia, for example the Barlow and Ortolani tests. To test for developmental hip dysplasia stand at the feet of baby and stabilize the pelvis with opposite side hand. Then flex the hip and knee, you are examining, 90 degrees. Then gently adduct the hip, push the femur posteriorly. Then abduct the hip feeling for a clunk or other subtle sense of abnormal motion. Other infant reflexes you can test for include rooting which is turning to the side a cheek is stroked, sucking and palmar grasp.

This is not complete coverage of the evaluation of a newborn, but it is enough to get you started thinking about how the physical examination of a new born baby is different from the physical examination of older patients.

Physical examination of a Young Child

The first thing to understand is that children are not simply small adults. Children have different needs. Children have different understanding of their problems. Children have different diseases and medical problems which vary with the child's age. I am not writing a textbook of pediatrics. My aim is to provide you with an introduction to the physical examination of a child, not a comprehensive textbook covering everything.

In a young child, particularly an anxious young child, I find it easier to perform the initial part of the exam while the parent is holding the child. This may also be true in starting your examination of a young child in pain. You can perform a much better initial exam with a quiet child in its parent's arms than with a screaming child lying on an examining table. In the young, not yet verbal child, I find this works well. Once the child settles down you begin your exam with gentle palpation of parts of the body which are clearly not likely to be involved or painful. You may place your hand gently on the child's back or hold their hand to get them used to you touching them without causing them pain. Then you can proceed to palpate other parts of the body. If there are fractures, for example of the tibia or clavicle or abdominal tenderness, this will manifest as tenderness as you carefully and systematically palpate various parts of the child's body.

*Case Study:*

*A six month old infant came into clinic when I was a medical student with bulging fontanels. The only symptom was a complaint by his mother of increased irritability. After detailed work up was unrevealing, the pediatrician took a more detailed history. Finally, the pediatrician discovered that the infant's mother was feeding her child calves liver every day because it was "healthy." Liver has large amounts of Vitamin A. This presentation was the result of hypervitaminosis A. An unusual cause of bulging fontanels. The bulging fontanels were the only abnormality on physical exam. The diagnosis could only be made by taking a careful, thorough and thoughtful medical history.*

In evaluating a non-verbal child with a limp or unwillingness to bear weight on a leg, you evaluate whether the child is willing to bear weight on the leg while kneeling or not. Unwillingness to bear weight on the knee of the involved side suggests a problem above the knee, usually femur or hip. Willingness to bear weight on the knee but not the foot suggests a problem in the lower leg, ankle or foot. Be aware that a child with multiple fractures or fractures of different ages on x-ray may be suffering abuse. Be aware that a child with bruising in multiple areas may be suffering abuse. Signs like this must not be ignored.

*Case Study:*

*A six month old baby came into my office due to refusal to move his left arm. There was tenderness over the humerus. X-rays showed a spiral fracture of the humerus. This is a common abuse fracture in the infant from twisting the arm. After detailed and determined questioning, the father admitted to twisting the baby's arm while angry. I reported this to the proper authorities and they began counseling and supervision of the family.*

*Case Study:*
*A three year old child was brought into my office due to refusal to put weight on his right leg. He would not put weight on his right knee either. When the child was distracted there was tenderness to deep palpation at the distal metaphysis of the right femur. No other anatomic structures were tender. X-rays were normal. Bone scan was positive for increased uptake in the distal metaphysis of the right femur. Diagnosis: hematogenous osteomyelitis. Treatment included immediate hospitalization and intravenous antibiotics with good result. Making the diagnosis required careful, thoughtful and systematic palpation of various anatomic structures in a protocol driven order.*

Note: In the absence of a clear, observed history of trauma and a presentation of refusal to bear weight with normal x-rays, work up for possible hematogenous osteomyelitis is mandatory. A delay in diagnosis is serious.

Part of the physical examination of a child is the correlation of height and weight with age. Abnormalities in following the normal growth curve need to be evaluated.

Any child with the spontaneous limp or limp after a reported minor injury needs to be evaluated. Many patients with diagnoses having nothing to do with trauma will present with a limp and will have a history of some minor trauma which is felt to be the cause. Don't be fooled by a history of minor trauma.

For the physical examination of a child with a limp: With the child supine and distracted, gentle log rolling of the uninvolved hip should not cause complaint. If performed on the symptomatic side it may cause pain. I usually perform log rolling by gently rolling the knee back and forth with my hand on the patella or lower thigh. I initially palpate the patella and thigh to ensure that they are not tender themselves. If log rolling is positive it suggests a problem with the hip, femur or knee. X-rays are mandatory. Diagnoses which may cause this include septic arthritis of the hip, hematogenous osteomyelitis, toxic synovitis of the hip, Legg-Calve-Perthes disease (avascular necrosis of the femoral head) and fracture of the femur in young children. In young teenagers, x-rays are necessary to evaluate the possibility of slipped capital femoral epiphysis.

Adult Physical Exam

Before I touch a patient, I have already observed how they sit, lie down, move and talk while I am taking their medical history. Depending on the medical history obtained and the initial observation, the physical examination will vary significantly.

For example, if the patient proves to be a remarkably poor historian, I may move directly to a quick cognitive status evaluation. If the patient seems almost sedated, I may look at the pupils for evidence of drug use. As I begin my examination, I talk with the patient touch them gently and palpate lightly areas which I do not expect to be tender. I wish the patient to get used to my touching. I wish to evaluate how the patient reacts to this light touching. Is the patient hyper-reactive? I am obtaining a base line of my patient's reaction to light palpation in non-tender areas.

Subjective vs objective findings

Before moving on to the physical examination in greater detail, let's touch on the difference between subjective and objective findings on the physical exam. Objective findings do not require any cooperation from the patient. Examples include the color of the skin, the appearance of skin lesions, heart sounds on auscultation, palpation of masses, testing for joint instability and a bone sticking out of the skin in a compound fracture.

*Case Study:*

*A patient was referred to my office with complaints of left arm pain. The imme-diate observational abnormality was generalized increased redness involving the entire left arm which I could see below the sleeve of the shirt. The right arm was normal color. My exam proceeded with removing the shirt to allow me to see the entire left arm. Thin circumferential bruising and indentation were seen in skin of the upper arm. With careful questioning my patient admitted that she was repeatedly binding her arm tightly. After determining I could find no other cause of her arm pain, I referred her for psychiatric evaluation and treatment. The increased redness of the left arm was an objective finding. The thin, circumferential bruising and indentation of the upper arm were objective findings even though medical history initially was not revealing.*

Subjective findings include evaluation of posture, gait, muscle strength, sensation including touch, smell, hearing, taste and touch and mental status responses.

Much of the physical examination is subjective. Even listening to the lungs may be subjective since the patient may not take a normal deep breath. Thus, it is important as an early part of every physical examination to determine a sense of a patient's cooperation and reliability. It is important to evaluate the presence or absence of symptom exaggeration and/or hypersensitivity. This is important in evaluating new patients; perhaps less so for well known, established patients.

For a general yearly physical examination you can examine in any order you choose. I think starting at the head and working downwards decreases the chance of skipping something. For a general yearly physical examination it is important to be thorough. I know of yearly exams in which clothes were not removed to look at the skin for skin cancers. I know of yearly physical exams in women in which the bra was not removed for a breast exam. I can go on. It is easy to get lazy and sloppy.

For a complaint specific examination, the exam will, of course, be more complaint centered. Thus, the physical examination for a complaint of chest pain will follow the cardiovascular and the pulmonary physical examinations discussed later. Similarly, the physical examination for shortness of breath would include the exam of both cardiovascular and pulmonary systems. A complaint of abdominal pain will at the minimum include the exam of the abdomen discussed later.

If I am performing a physical examination for a complaint related to the upper extremity, I initially ask the patient to raise her arms over her head. Obviously, this is skipped if there is obvious significant trauma to the upper arm. Does the patient move her arms up over her head normally? Is there limited motion? Does it appear painful? Does the patient appear to make a normal, honest effort? Is there any sense of exaggeration or unusual affected movement? I am performing a quick check for shoulder range of motion and deltoid function while at the same time evaluating the patient for evidence of anxiety, hypersensitivity or exaggeration of symptoms. If I detect a sense of hypersensitivity or exaggeration of symptoms, my examination immediately shifts gears to evaluate that possibility further.

My history should have already covered the question of possible third party liability. This is perhaps more important in orthopedics than other specialties but issues of third party liability may pop up in almost any specialty. So, in my history I ask after trauma and what the patient thinks may have caused the symptoms. If there is any question of third party liability, I take a more detailed causation history and perform a more careful physical examination because I understand that in a year or three I may be asked to testify under oath regarding my history and physical examination. I wish to ensure that I have not omitted anything important. The same is true if I evaluate a patient for whom there may be malpractice issues from past medical treatment.

In children and teenagers, further history may occasionally be important to pick up school aversion due to bullying or other causes. This questioning needs to occur with the child or teenager alone without parents present. I have not seen this often, but I picked up a few cases in my career of school age children with complaints preventing them from attending school with minimal findings on physical exam.

# CHAPTER EIGHT:

# Palpation

Before moving on to the physical examination of specific systems or parts of the body, I wish to devote an entire chapter to the "art" and the "science" of palpation as a part of the physical examination on its own. I think that insufficient time was spent discussing and teaching palpation in my training. This was a skill I developed over time more by teaching myself than by actual instruction. Palpation is a skill which develops with thoughtful experience. I wish to discuss techniques of using palpation and the need for careful and thoughtful palpation of anatomic structures and the need for thoroughness in palpation of anatomic structures.

Many of the patients with missed diagnoses, I saw in my career, occurred because of sloppy, inadequate, unfocused, unsystematic palpation of anatomic structures by other medical providers. Palpation is a more important part of the physical examination of the musculoskeletal system than that of the other systems excepting perhaps the abdominal examination. Proper palpation is key to a careful and thorough physical examination of the musculoskeletal system. Not so much with the other systems. Perhaps that is why palpation is poorly understood and poorly taught by non-orthopedic surgeons.

*Case Study:*

*A 53 year old woman comes to a suburban emergency room complaining of left shoulder pain. The emergency room physician performs a cursory exam and diagnoses bursitis of the shoulder. He administers a cortisone shot. The patient returns to the same emergency room a few hours later complaining of increasingly severe pain. By protocol, all returns to this emergency room are supposed to be seen by a physician. In this situation, the patient is seen by a physician's assistant. The physician's assistant assumes the patient is "hysterical." He performs a limited physical exam and sends her out.*

*This woman is an old patient of mine. I know her well. I have seen her before for a number of orthopedic problems. She is not a histrionic patient. She calls me a few hours after her second discharge from the emergency room, frantic with severe shoulder pain. I tell her to come straight to the emergency room. I tell her that I will meet her there. Half an hour later, I see a woman in serious distress, in severe pain, sitting on an examining table. I begin the palpation part of my physical exam with gentle palpation of the superficial anatomy of the shoulder. I follow my specific protocol for palpation of the shoulder. I palpate the sterno-clavicular joint. No reaction. I palpate the clavicle. No reaction. I palpate the acromio-clavicular joint. Chandelier sign! She rises up off of the table rapidly and impressively. I diagnose septic arthritis, that is, a bacterial infection of the acromio-clavicular joint. I treat her with surgical drainage and antibiotics. Postoperative cultures were positive for staphylococcus. The only time in my career, I saw septic arthritis of the acromio-clavicular joint.*

*Why present this case to you, the reader?*

*Why was the diagnosis missed by the emergency room physician at the initial visit and later missed by the physician's assistant at the return visit?*

*The failure of these two medical providers to palpate the specific anatomic structures of the shoulder following a thoughtful protocol was the reason this rare, and I do mean rare, diagnosis was missed initially. Neither of these medical providers utilized a specific detailed protocol for examining the shoulder which included the palpation of precise and specific anatomic structures. Neither of these medical providers utilized a specific detailed protocol for examining the shoulder which included specific palpation of the acromio-clavicular joint.*

Your need to establish for yourself a specific physical examination protocol for how you examine each and every part of the body. Your protocol does not need to be my protocol. As you go through your training sort out what physical examination protocols you think are best.

**To the extent your examination protocol is thorough**

**To the extent your examination protocol is complete**

**To the extent that you <u>always</u>, and I mean <u>always</u>, follow your examination protocol,**

**you will be less likely to miss important findings.**

*Case Study:*
*I have just entered the United States Army as an orthopedic surgeon and have just come to the orthopedic clinic to see my first patients. The sergeant in charge of the clinic tells me that my first patient is a malingerer, who has been hanging around the clinic for six months and does not want to work. I see the patient and take his history. He was involved in an accident which was not his fault. The army truck he was driving was hit head on and he hit his hand on the steering wheel. He has had continued pain with tight gripping for the six months since the accident. He states that he cannot drive a heavy truck because of this pain. He has been seen by two previous orthopedic surgeons in the army orthopedic clinic. Both were graduates of the Harvard Combined Orthopedic Residency program. Both entered the service in the Berry Plan. Neither of the two previous examining orthopedic surgeons found anything abnormal on physical exam.*

*Having been told that the patient is a malingerer, I perform a somewhat perfunctory physical exam and send him away.*

And. Yet! And. Yet! And. Yet!

*Suddenly! I realize that I have failed to perform my usual complete proto-col-driven wrist and hand physical exam. I dash out of my office and call the patient back into my examination room. Then, I carefully perform my custom-ary, complete wrist and hand examination following my personal wrist and hand examination protocol. One small part of my wrist and hand examina-tion protocol is palpation of the proximal ulnar palm side of the hand over a structure called the hook of the hamate. This patient's exam has been normal, physiologic and non-histrionic, so far. I palpate many specific anatomical parts of the wrist and hand and find no tenderness. I palpate the hook of the hamate. He complains of pain.*

*X-rays are normal. Fractures of the hook of the hamate do not usually show up on routine x-rays. These fractures are "hidden" on routine x-rays. I order a CT scan of the wrist which shows a non-union of a fracture of the hook of the hamate. I cast this patient for six weeks. The non-union heals. He returns to work without complaint.*

*The correct diagnosis was missed in this patient by two Harvard trained ortho-pedic surgeons prior to my exam. The wrist/hand physical examination protocol for these two orthopedic surgeons did not include palpation of the hook of the hamate. Thus, they both missed the diagnosis.*

**I present this case to emphasize the need for you, the reader, to develop a complete, thorough protocol for how you examine each and every part of the body. I present this case to emphasize the need for you, the reader, to develop a complete, thorough protocol for how you palpate each and every part of the body. I, also, emphasize the need for you to perform your complete and thorough examination each and every time.**

*In this particular case, I <u>almost, almost, almost</u> missed the diagnosis, because I initially failed to perform my usual, complete, protocol-driven examination of the wrist and hand.*

Of the five senses: taste, smell, sight, hearing and touch, we seem to utilize sight and hearing the most and become dependent on them. Although we use touch to pick up a glass and hold the glass without dropping it from an early age, we do not develop the sense of touch as we grow older as much as we might. Any practice using our brain, spinal cord and peripheral nerves, improves the function of that activity. An oenophile may develop her ability to detect subtle differences in wines which she could not detect before training. A gymnast develops increased balance and the ability to "know" where she is in the air with continued training. Similarly, a beginning medical clinician is able with thoughtful practice to develop and improve the use of touch and palpation in physical examination.

Depending on what you are palpating you may utilize an extremely light touch, a medium touch or a deep touch.

*Case Study:*
*A patient was referred to me by the workers compensation insurance company. By history a weight fell on the back of this patient's hand. He had not worked for six months because of continued pain in his hand. Covert video surveillance was obtained by the insurance company. The insurance company was convinced that this patient was faking his pain. The covert surveillance video showed the patient helping a friend move heavy objects onto the back of a pickup truck. At one point the patient stops and shakes his hand for ten seconds. He then resumes helping his friend. His treating orthopedic surgeon found nothing and assumed he was malingering. The insurance company sent the patient to me for an independent medical evaluation.*

*At my evaluation, this patient complains of pain on the dorsum of his third metacarpal phalangeal joint. He is quite specific about where he feels his pain.*

*He points to one specific point of maximum pain. This does not seem like a fraudulent complaint. His complaints do not seem exaggerated. His physical examination initially seems normal. He demonstrates full, painless, smooth motion of the fingers. I do not sense symptom magnification or other non-physiologic behavior in my examination.*

*Clearly, the patient felt something when he was helping his friend move. Images on the video clearly showed him stopping and shaking his hand. There was no sense that he knew he was being watched and no sense that he was exaggerating his symptoms on the video.*

*I am sure something is "there." I just can't find it. I do not palpate a mass. I examine more carefully. I palpate the dorsum of his third metacarpal phalangeal joint as gently as I can, while he flexes and extends his fingers. I do this with my eyes closed and using as gentle palpation as I can. I detect a most, subtle rubbing, vibratory sensation under my palpating fingers on the dorsum of the metacarpal phalangeal joint as he flexes and extends his fingers. Something deep under the extensor hood is rubbing as he flexes and extends his fingers.*

*I suspect a benign mass, likely a lipoma is present under the extensor hood at the joint. Never seen one before. Never seen one since. I recommend surgical exploration. The insurance company approves. At surgical exploration, I find a flat lipoma under the extensor digitorum communis tendon of the middle finger at the extensor hood and excise it. After being out of work for six months, this patient returns to work three weeks after my surgery. The treating orthopedic surgeon missed this subtle physical finding. Granted, this was an extremely subtle finding on exam. His treating orthopedic surgeon's evaluation was not sufficiently thoughtful and careful to detect this.*

This particular case required exquisitely light palpation with my eyes closed over the area in question as the patient moved his finger. By closing my eyes, I enhanced the sensitivity of my light touch palpation. This allowed me to appreciate the sense of subtle vibration which indicated something was rubbing abnormally under my palpating fingers.

*Case Study:*

*A patient with right shoulder pain is referred to me for an Independent Medical Examination. This is a work related injury and the Workers' Compensation Insurance Company wants my opinion regarding what if anything is wrong with this patient who has been out of work for four months. The treating orthopedic surgeon is requesting permission to perform right shoulder arthroscopy to try to determine the cause of this patient's pain. By history from the patient, a heavy weight fell on her shoulder while at work. She has been unable to work since that time.*

*The shoulder is normal to observation and palpation of specific anatomical structures. I find no areas of tenderness. As part of my routine upper extremity muscle testing, I have the patient push with her right hand against my left hand while I palpate the right scapula. The right scapula wings out dramatically. The patient has a long thoracic nerve palsy which results in paralysis of the serratus anterior muscle, which holds the scapula against the thoracic cage. Long thoracic nerve palsy may be caused by a heavy weight falling on the top of the shoulder. Shoulder arthroscopy will not help the nerve palsy. The treating orthopedic surgeon missed this diagnosis over four months of treatment because his shoulder examination protocol did not include testing for weakness of the serratus anterior muscle. The treating orthopedic surgeon missed this diagnosis because his shoulder examination protocol was incomplete.*

I am including in this chapter on palpation a number of case studies in which the original medical provider missed the diagnosis due to a failure to perform a sufficiently complete, thorough, anatomic palpation of the involved part of the body. You may argue that these diagnoses were rare and thus easy to miss. I agree. They were rare and easy to miss.

I recognize that I am being arrogant in this discussion. What "physical examination behaviors" of mine allowed me to make these diagnoses which were missed by other medical providers? I submit that my physical examinations including my palpations are more thorough, more complete and more carefully anatomic than the average medical provider. My physical examinations and my anatomic palpations are protocol driven to minimize the risk of my missing something.

I confess to being preachy. I confess to hectoring you. I confess that I am arrogant that I made so many diagnoses which were missed by others. Let me ask you a question, "If my arrogance is deserved, what physical examination behaviors of mine led to my ability to make more diagnoses, more quickly than most?" I repeat: My physical examinations including my palpations are more thorough, more complete and more carefully anatomic than the average medical provider. My physical examinations and my anatomic palpations are protocol driven to minimize the risk of my missing something.

**I am hoping to convince you to carefully and thoroughly develop your own complete and thorough protocol driven physical examinations.**

Let's continue my palpation discussion. With medium palpation you can determine the character, the quality, the consistency of masses. What do I mean by the consistency of masses? Some masses are fluid filled and demonstrate fluctuance. Some masses are clearly firm or hard. Some masses are hard enough that they feel like and are bony protrusions. Rare masses have a woody, dense spongey feeling.

As noted before, sensations are hard to describe.

*Case Study:*
*A 32 year old man comes into my office complaining of a mass on the dorsal radial aspect of his hand which is not tender. The mass has been slowly increasing in size over several months. The mass is irregular on medium palpation and*

*feels woody and densely spongey. Here, again, is where the patient's history and the physical exam intersect, intermingle and intertwine with each other. With my physical findings, I take a more detailed "hand injury" history. Months previously, he scraped the back of his hand on a pier in a harbor. As a result of the history of injury and the physical examination findings of a woody, dense, spongey feeling of this mass, I suspect an infection with either a fungus or an atypical mycobacterium.*

*Surgical exploration and excisional biopsy were performed. Prolonged culture in special culture medium for fungus and atypical mycobacterium grew out an atypical mycobacterium, mycobacterium marinum. The "simple" palpation in my office alerted me to this possible diagnosis. Why was this important? If I fail to recognize this preoperatively, I will not obtain the proper, special cultures. If I fail to obtain the proper special cultures, routine cultures will show no growth. The infection will continue. Diagnosis will be delayed. The patient will be improperly treated.*

*In this case, I consulted with an infectious disease specialist preoperatively. Thus, the proper, special fungal and mycobacterial culture media were available in the operating room for immediate culture. Anti-mycobacterial medicine was begun immediately after surgery and the patient recovered without reinfection. This is an example of the importance of a careful and thoughtful physical examination, the importance of proper palpation and the importance of acting on the information obtained.*

When examining the abdomen, deep palpation is used to exam for increased size of the liver and spleen. Deep palpation is also used when testing for rebound tenderness. Deep palpation of the abdomen is also used to look for abdominal aortic aneurysms.

*Case Study:*

*A 63 year old man was referred by his internist to the office of an orthopedic surgeon, one of my partners, complaining of intense, tearing pain in his back. Examination of the mid and low back was unremarkable. Due to the negative back exam and the character of the pain, the orthopedic surgeon extended his examination and performed an abdominal examination which included deep palpation of the abdomen. On deep palpation of the abdomen the orthopedic surgeon noted a large pulsatile mass. He called an ambulance and had the patient transferred urgently to the nearest emergency room for emergency surgery for a dissecting abdominal aortic aneurysm, thereby saving the patient's life.*

*Yes, the abdominal examination is, at times, a critical part of the orthopedic examination.*

*Yes, the abdominal examination is, at times, a critical part of the examination of the spine.*

*I repeat: Physical examination of the low back and spine, at times, needs to include an abdominal examination.*

**An abdominal examination should be part of any back exam which does not provide confirming physical findings.**

**An abdominal examination should be part of any back exam for which the complaints of back pain are not the common type of complaints.**

Palpation of Masses

When palpating masses, you are evaluating at times whether there is a mass present or not. If there is a mass, what size is it? Is the mass moveable or fixed? Is the mass hard or soft? If hard, is the mass soft tissue hard or boney hard? Is the mass solid or fluctuant? Is the mass a smooth lump or is does the mass have an irregular shape? Is there more than one mass? What is the location of the mass? Does the mass trans-illuminate? Is the mass tender to palpation? Is the mass warm or red?

When you palpate a mass, there are numerous characteristics which may be defined and described.

Masses which are small, soft and moveable are likely to be benign. Masses which are large, firm and fixed are likely to be malignant. Masses which are warm, tender and reddish are likely to be infected abscesses. Masses which trans-illuminate are fluid filled.

Over my many years of training and practice I have come to appreciate the use of the technique of palpation as a more subtle, nuanced procedure than I first thought. Palpation may involve deep, pressured probing. Consider the abdominal exam. You press deeply and then ask the patient to inhale deeply when palpating for possible hepatomegaly and splenomegaly. You also palpate deeply and then release quickly looking for rebound tenderness which indicates irritation of peritoneum or peritonitis.

Palpation needs to be as soft and as gentle as is possible to touch someone while attempting to sense some abnormal feeling as the patient moves under the gentle palpation. Palpation needs to be as soft and as gentle as is possible when trying to determine whether a small subtle mass is present or not.

A fluid filled mass behaves differently on examination than a solid mass. Common benign fluid filled masses are ganglions which are most common on the dorsum of the wrist. They also occur commonly at the volar radial wrist, at the level of the A1 pulley of the hand flexor tendon sheaths, at the first dorsal extensor compartment and at the dorsum of the distal interphalangeal joints of the fingers and thumb. When they occur on a tendon sheath they may be called ganglions of tendon sheath. When they occur at the dorsum of the distal interphalangeal joint they may be called mucous cysts.

Fluid filled cysts may present with fluctuance on exam unless they are small and fixed to a tendon sheath. What is fluctuance? Imagine you are blind-folded and place both of your hands on a water balloon on a table. If I push on the water balloon you will feel a fluid impulse with the fingers of both of your hands. If you push in on the water balloon with one hand you will feel a fluid wave with the fingers of the other hand.

The fluid wave you feel with one of your examining hands on the water balloon is fluctuance. In firm fluid filled cysts determining fluctuance requires a subtle touch and examination. Ganglions will often demonstrate fluctuance with gentle palpation of the fingers of the other hand following pressure applied with the fingers of the first hand. Ganglions of tendon sheath are often small and firm and you will not be able to detect fluctuance on exam. When examining for subtle abnormalities, I find that closing my eyes, in order to decrease other sensory input, allows me to perceive subtle cues and clues of sensation which I might not otherwise perceive.

The sensation of fluctuance is used in the examination of joints for effusions. In examining the wrist joint for a dorsal ganglion, grasp the wrist gently with both hands with one thumb dorsal radial and one thumb dorsal ulnar over the wrist joint. Then alternatively push gently with each thumb feeling with the other thumb for the presence or absence of a subtle fluid wave. In the knee with one hand push down gently just above the patella to compress the suprapatellar pouch. With the other hand feel gently with the thumb on the medial or lateral joint line and the fingers on the opposite side of the knee at the joint line. Then alternately push down on the suprapatellar pouch or inward at the medial and lateral joint line feeling for a sense of a fluid wave with the fingers which are not pushing. Similar examination maneuvers may be used for examining for joint effusions for the elbow, metacarpal phalangeal joint and ankle joint. Common fluctuant swellings about the knee include bursal effusions anterior to the patella (patellar bursa) and anterior to the tibial tubercle (prepatellar bursa). A common swelling posterior to the elbow occurs in the olecranon bursa. These bursal effusions may be determined during physical examination by testing for fluctuance.

Transillumination of masses

Testing for possible transillumination of a mass helps when trying to determine if a mass is fluid filled. I find using a small pen light works well. A common mass is a ganglion of the dorsum of a wrist. Fluctuance is often felt. Transillumination confirms that the mass is fluid filled. You see the light spread through the fluid. Ganglions may appear anywhere in the body. Transillumination again will test whether the mass is fluid filled.

There is a rare mass called a glomus tumor which often arises in the nailbed of a finger. It may present with complaints of irritating pain in the distal finger in the presence of a normal physical exam. In reported series of glomus tumors, the average delay between onset of symptoms and diagnosis is often around seven years. A rare tumor. I saw about eight in my career as a hand and orthopedic surgeon. Some glomus tumors may be diagnosed by seeing a dark spot under the fingernail upon transillumination of the fingertip. If the average gap between onset of symptoms and diagnosis is seven years, think how many medical providers saw each patient, missed the diagnosis and discharged the patient as histrionic. Thus, any patient who complains of fingertip pain with an otherwise normal exam should be evaluated with transillumination of the nail bed. Normal transillumination of the nail bed does not completely rule out a glomus tumor.

# CHAPTER NINE:

# The neurologic examination

In the next few chapters, I discuss symptom specific and part of the body specific physical examinations. I shall begin by discussing the physical examination oriented to specific physiologic systems. I start with the neurologic examination. There is no specific reason for the order of systems I discuss.

The examination of the neurological system includes the central nervous system and the peripheral nervous system. The central nervous system includes evaluation of consciousness and/or mental status, the cranial nerves, and the spinal cord. The peripheral nervous system includes the evaluation of the peripheral motor nerves, the peripheral sensory nerves and the mixed motor and sensory peripheral nerves. For my purposes, I am categorizing the physical examination for possible primary myopathies under the neurologic examination. Evaluating the differential diagnosis of muscle weakness always involves an examination of the neurological system. The extent of any physical examination of each depends on the patient's complaints and the purpose of the examination.

Alteration of mental status may be due to some primary brain malfunction or from an external cause such as drugs, medication side effects and trauma. Alteration in function of the cranial nerves may be centrally caused as happens with tumors or peripheral such as acoustical neuromas or tumors which press on the optic chiasm. Alterations in the function of the spinal cord may come from viral or immune effects such as shingles and Parsonage Turner Syndrome, from tumors, infections and injury among other causes. Alterations in the function of the peripheral nervous system may come from primary neuropathies, primary myopathies, combined neuropathies and trauma.

In trauma there will be a defined and specific loss of nerve function. There will be a pure sensory loss if a peripheral sensory nerve is damaged such as a laceration of a digital nerve in the finger or from pressure as in meralgia paresthetica. There will be pure muscle weakness if a pure motor nerve is injured as in the anterior interosseous syndrome in which chronic pressure on a terminal branch of the median nerve causes specific muscle weakness. There will be a mixed sensory and motor loss of function if a mixed nerve is injured. This is seen in carpal tunnel syndrome, cubital tunnel syndrome, brachial plexus injuries and lacerations of more proximal nerves.

If there is any question that a patient is faking an unconscious state, you can lift up one arm and hand and place the arm and hand over the patient's face. In an unconscious patient, the hand will drop onto the face. In a patient faking an unconscious state the hand and arm will often "strangely" fail to flop onto the patient's face.

Mental Status

First: Is the patient conscious or unconscious. If unconscious the issues of airway, breathing and heart function take emergent precedence. Further discussion here assumes that those issues have been evaluated and treated as appropriate.

Unconscious

A determination of the level of consciousness and the cause of unconscious-ness are a priority. If there is any question of drug overdose, particularly

narcotics, the immediate administration of Narcan is indicated. Any unconscious patient should have a blood sugar drawn STAT and be given an amp of
D50W because of the possibility of insulin shock. I am going to move beyond
the emergency evaluation and treatment.

*Case Study:*
*I am on the neurosurgery service and am called to see a patient who has suffered*
*a gunshot wound to the face. The patient is unconscious, spontaneously breath-*
*ing with a normal heart rate. There is a small entry wound on the front of the*
*nose. The senior neurosurgery resident and I roll the patient over to look for an*
*exit wound. There is no exit wound.*

*The neurosurgery resident and I wish to establish the level of consciousness.*
*There is no withdrawal response to pinching skin on the lower leg or arms. The*
*patient's pupils are fixed and dilated. The pupils do not respond to light. This*
*indicates a lack of function of the third cranial nerve, the oculomotor nerve.*
*We next perform the Doll's Eyes Reflex, also known as the oculocephalic reflex.*
*The oculocephalic reflex tests cranial nerves 3, 6 and 8. This test should only*
*be performed if there is assurance that the cervical spine is stable. Holding the*
*eyelids up the head is rapidly rotated to one side. If the test is positive the eyes*
*rotate opposite to the direction of motion and remain facing forward. If the eyes*
*rotate with the head the test is negative. If the test is negative there is dysfunc-*
*tion in one or more of the pathways which modulate this reflex. In our patient,*
*the Doll's Eyes Reflex indicate a lack of brain stem function.*

*Next, we test Caloric Stimulation. We pour warm water into each ear sequen-*
*tially. This tests the acoustic nerve or 8ᵗʰ cranial nerve. If the nerve is working*
*then the eyes will rotate with nystagmus toward the side of the warm water.*
*In this patient, caloric stimulation demonstrated complete lack of function of*
*the 8ᵗʰ cranial nerve.*

*The neurosurgery resident demonstrates clearly and quickly the complete*
*absence of brain stem function, that is, he demonstrates convincingly that*

*this patient is brain dead. There is a small entrance wound on the front of the nose and no exit wound. Presumably, the bullet has entered the skull and spun around inside the skull. We call for portable x-ray to find the location of the bullet. While waiting for portable x-ray to arrive our patient suddenly blinks his eyes and wakes up with normal mental status. X-rays, when obtained, show the bullet lodged in the mastoid process on one side. Presumably, the shock wave of the bullet's passage caused a temporary loss of brain stem function. This unusual presentation probably resulted from the fact that the bullet was low velocity .22 caliber.*

I present this case in order to introduce you to tests for cranial nerve and brain stem function. I am not presenting a complete rendition of the examination of the comatose patient. I am merely giving you an introduction. Detailed evaluation of the comatose patient is beyond the scope of this book.

There exists a rating or scoring of depth of coma called the Glascow Coma Score which rates eye, verbal and motor responses to stimuli on a scale from 3 to 15. Discussing this rating system is beyond the scope of this book.

Conscious Patient Mental Status Evaluation, aka Cognitive Status Evaluation

For the quick, quick evaluation, you ask the patient, "What is your name? Where are you? What is the date? Who is the president of the United States?" When should you use this? Far more often than you think you should.

I ask these questions of all of my elderly hip fracture patients? A surprising number do not answer all four questions correctly. I am not concerned if a retired patient is off by a day or two or struggles to figure out precisely what number date it is. A wrong month, a wrong year, a wrong president, a blank response indicate a concerning degree of cognitive impairment. Follow up of a response concerning for cognitive impairment involves determining the severity of the impairment and the question whether the impairment is known or unknown by family and primary care physician and whether it is recent or long standing.

A slightly longer cognitive status evaluation is called the Mini Mental Status Examination or the Folstein Test. This is a 30 point test which does not require special equipment. The testing involves knowing the time and place, repeating named prompts, serial 7s, spelling the word "world" backwards, naming three objects and asking for their recall five minutes later, naming objects like a pencil and watch, repeating back a phrase and copying on paper a diagram of two intersecting pentagons. I am not covering the precise details of the Folstein Test. The details are available elsewhere. Another test of cognitive status I have read about but have not used is to ask a patient to draw a clock face showing a specified time. This simple test may pick up subtle cognitive abnormalities. I have not gone into these tests in detail. My purpose is to give you an introduction to how you may quickly evaluate a patient's cognitive status.

I suggest you use the quick, quick person, place, time, president mini evaluation more often than you think you should. You will pick up occasional patients with more cognitive impairment than you expect.

Tests of Sensation

I have previously discussed the difference between subjective and objective parts of the physical examination. Tests of sensation are completely, totally and thoroughly subjective, except possibly when examining for response to pain in a comatose patient. Patients must be willing and able to cooperate. This requires a fair degree of cognitive function. In third party liability situations attempts at symptom magnification may occur.

I am not covering tests of taste and smell. These are specialized tests which are beyond the scope of this book.

Sight; Eyes

Visual acuity is usually tested with charts and or machines. Detailed testing of visual acuity is beyond the scope of this book. Similarly, tests for color blindness are beyond the scope of this book. Simple and quick evaluation of the eyes include observation. Do the eyes look normal? Are the eyes bulging called exophthalmos or proptosis? Do you see sclera (the white) above the iris? Hyperthyroidism is a common cause. A tumor behind the eye is another. Are the irises white or yellowish? Is the pupil size symmetric? Asymmetric pupils are called anisocoria. Some people have asymmetric pupils with no other serious cause. If noted, a patient should be referred to an ophthalmologist for further evaluation. Do the pupils react to light and accommodation? Are the extraocular motions full?

A quick test for field of vision. Have the patient stare at your eyes. Look at the patient to ensure the patient continues to stare at your eyes. Hold up your hands a little above your head and to either side. Ask the patient to tell you when she sees your finger move. Then intermittently move the index finger of one or the other hand. Similarly, hold your hands out to the side at waist level and do the same with moving your fingers sequentially and asking the patient to tell you when you move your fingers. Obviously, this test will not pick up subtle areas of loss of field of vision. It will pick up major quadrant losses of field of vision.

Hearing

Detailed tests of hearing are performed by audiologists. Gross tests for hearing in each ear may be performed by asking a patient to close her eyes and tell you when and if she hears you rubbing two fingers together just outside her ear.

If there is concern regarding the truthfulness of a patient's claimed hearing loss of one ear, you can place a vibrating tuning fork against the skull near the "affected" ear and ask the patient if he hears anything. An answer of "No" will indicate symptom magnification since bone conduction will carry the vibration sound to the opposite ear. The use of a tuning fork on the skull may help differentiate between hearing loss from air conduction and nerve conduction.

Touch

The evaluation of light touch sensation is an important part of the evaluation of partial and complete spinal cord injuries. For example, in the Brown-Sequard Syndrome, there is injury to one half of the spinal cord resulting in weakness or paralysis of one half of the body below the injury in the spinal cord and loss of sensation in the other half of the body.

Evaluation of light touch sensation is also an important part of the evaluation of possible peripheral nerve injuries. The more localized the area of decreased sensation or loss of sensation the more peripheral the nerve injury. The more diffuse the area of decreased sensation or loss of sensation, the more proximal the nerve injury. There is always the possibility of more than one area of nerve injury.

*Case Study:*
*A motorcycle policeman came into my office with the complaint of numbness and decreased feeling in the lateral, distal lower leg, lateral ankle and lateral foot. This was an old patient of mine. I knew him well. Physical examination disclosed normal motor exam in detail for the lower extremity and decreased light touch sensation in the lateral lower leg and dorsal lateral foot. Tapping around the lateral, lower leg, I found one specific place where the Tinel's sign caused a feeling of numbness and tingling radiating to the lateral foot. There was no evidence of a recent or old skin break. Clearly this was an isolated, neuropraxia of the sensory nerve innervating the distal lateral leg, ankle and lateral foot.*

*But why?*

*This is a distinctly unusual place to have a neuropraxia of a sensory nerve. Here, I mention observation again. I have seen my patient a number of times in the past, always wearing old, loved, well used motorcycle boots which were part of his uniform. This time I see new boots off to the side and ask to see them. These new boots have a single crease on the outside where the inside of the crease presents a fairly sharp edge to the lateral aspect of my patient's distal leg. Cause found. Chronic pressure from this single crease in the new motorcycle boots.*

*My initial advice is to go back to the old boots. My patient states that is not possible. He is under orders to wear the new, better looking boots. My treatment then consists of advice to wear a bandage under the crease to distribute the pressure from the crease. I also recommend massage and manipulation of the boots to soften them to eliminate the one distinct crease.*

This was a case of a neuropraxia of a pure sensory nerve far distal with a small limited area of loss of light touch sensation. Back to observation. If I don't look carefully for a cause of the neuropraxia, if I don't observe the crease in the new motorcycle boots, I will not figure out the cause of the neuropraxia and I will not successfully treat my patient.

*Case Study:*

*A 45 year old slightly obese man came into my office complaining of numbness of the anterior and lateral left thigh. He did not complain of pain. Motor exam of the lower extremity was normal in detail. The joints of the lower extremity had full, painless range of motion. There was an area of the anterior and lateral thigh of decreased light touch sensation. This is meralgia parenthetica. Meralgia paresthetica is caused by pressure on the lateral femoral cutaneous nerve. This nerve passes from the groin to the upper thigh and neuropraxia of that nerve may be caused by pressure from the inguinal ligament.*

*I have read about meralgia paresthetica causing pain and requiring treatment. In my personal experience, patients described their symptoms as mild and required no specific treatment. Some of my patients were obese. The numbness often went away after a year or two. In my personal experience I found this in patients often as the result of a careful sensory examination, although my patient had not complained of thigh numbness. In my experience, reassurance was the only treatment necessary.*

Here is another case of a neuropraxia of a pure sensory nerve which is relatively distal and results in a small limited area of loss of light touch sensation.

*Case Study:*
*A patient was referred to my office with complaints of weakness of his right hand and numbness and loss of feeling in his ring and little finger. First, observation. The patient was sitting with a typical ulnar claw hand. At rest, the ring and little finger were extended at the metacarpal phalangeal joints and flexed at the proximal interphalangeal joints. There was obvious atrophy of the intrinsic muscles of the hand. The spaces between the metacarpals were concave. This is the immediate sitting across from the patient observation. Examination disclosed absent sensation of the little finger, the ulnar side of the ring finger and the ulnar side of the hand. There was also complete absence of motor function of all of the ulnar nerve innervated muscles in the hand. There were no skin breaks or history of trauma.*

*This presentation is consistent with loss of function of the ulnar nerve somewhere below the elbow and above Guyon's canal. The ulnar nerve at the elbow and at Guyon's canal were normal to light palpation and the Tinel's sign was negative for both nerves. Nerve conduction velocity studies including an inching study along the forearm suggested that the defect in nerve conduction was approximately two inches proximal to Guyon's canal. There is nothing two inches proximal to Guyon's canal anatomically which can compress the ulnar nerve. I considered the possibility of a nerve tumor. I repeated the nerve conduction studies. The new studies again showed a conduction block two inches above Guyon's Canal. MRI scan did not show a mass or other abnormality in the nerve.*

*I surgically explored the ulnar nerve and found a 2 mm thick longitudinal wisp of abnormal tissue crossing the ulnar nerve two inches proximal to Guyon's canal. There was no indentation in the ulnar nerve. Careful exploration disclosed nothing else abnormal. I cut this wisp of tissue and closed the wound discouraged that I had not found the cause of the neuropraxia. In the recovery room, or I suppose I should say, in the post anesthesia care unit the patient demonstrated immediate complete recovery of nerve function. It is rare to see such dramatic results immediately following surgery. That thin little wisp of abnormal tissue which was not even making a dent in the edge of the nerve was applying just enough pressure to stop all function of the ulnar nerve without causing obvious gross physical damage to the nerve.*

Precise light touch sensation evaluation involves the determination of two point discrimination (2PD). This is only used for evaluating fingertip touch sensation. The fingertips have significantly greater numbers and density of touch sensor organs than anywhere else on the body.

To test 2PD you need a device which has two tips whose distance apart you can vary. Such instruments are available for purchase. The quick and easy way follows. Take a paper clip. Unbend all of the bends until the paper clip is as straight as you can make it. Then bend the paper clip in the middle so that the two tips are the same length and near each other. Now bend each half in its middle at a right angle to the previous bend. You have just manufactured a two point discrimination device and it didn't cost you anything. It is also available for free any time you have a paper clip available. With a ruler adjust the bends and the angles so that the tips measure 5 mm apart. You do need a ruler with millimeter measurements. You can then adjust the paper clip tips to the distance apart you wish to use in your two point discrimination evaluation.

Try this experiment on yourself. With your eyes closed, touch the two tips which are five millimeters apart gently on one of your fingertips. You should be able to feel two tips. For comparison, with your eyes closed touch the two tips to your proximal volar forearm. You should be unable to distinguish the two tips. This experiment will give you a sense of how sensitive your finger tips are.

When testing a patient for 2PD have the patient look away or cover the testing tips with your other hand so that the patient is unable to see if you are touching with one or two tips. You then randomly test by touching the patient's fingertip with one or two tips of the measuring device varying the distance between the two tips. The minimum distance a patient can distinguish whether she is being touched with one or two tips is often 5 mm. Occasional people are able to distinguish a 4 mm separation of the two tips.

A patient unable to distinguish tips 10 mm or more apart has no useful sensation of the finger. In the situation of a lacerated finger, hand or arm, greater than 10 mm 2PD suggests a nerve is cut or not functioning. Distinguishing 7-8mm but not less consistently suggests partial nerve function. 5 mm is normal nerve function.

In any acute care situation with an upper extremity laceration or puncture wound, two point discrimination should be performed and documented for both sides of all five digits. Missed nerve lacerations are common. I repeat, missed nerve lacerations are common. I repeat, missed nerve lacerations are common. Nerve lacerations are missed because of a failure to perform careful two point discrimination testing of all five digits.

Vibration sensation testing, temperature testing, sharp/dull testing, smooth/rough testing and stereognosis (position sense) are often used in detailed neurological evaluations. Detailed neurological exams are beyond the scope of this book. I use a few of these in other situations.

I frequently test position sense of the big toe when a patient has his eyes closed. I do this as a quick test for possible peripheral neuropathy. Peripheral neuropathy is common in the older population and seen occasionally in younger patients. It is seen more commonly in diabetics. Position sense of the big toe is a quick, quick method of looking for evidence of significant peripheral neuropathy Big toe position sense should be tested for any patient with a history of falls or multiple fractures. Big toe position sense should be tested regularly in all older patients. I tested big toe position sense in all of my adult patients who fell and fractured a bone.

Peripheral neuropathy is a major risk factor in falls. In patients with peripheral neuropathy the brain does not receive sufficient leg position sense information to maintain position and balance consistently. If peripheral neuropathy is found, patients should be evaluated for treatable causes of the neuropathy. If no medically treatable cause is found, then treatment with advice regarding use of canes and walkers to prevent further falls is indicated.

Sharp/dull and rough/smooth discrimination is often used in evaluating patient's recovering from the repair of nerve lacerations. Gentle palpation of the skin is also useful in evaluating nerve injuries. The skin of a fingertip will feel dry and smooth if there is no innervation of the skin due to the lack of innervation of the sweat glands. A normal fingertip has more resistance to lateral stroking across the fingertip due to the increased moisture on the tip of the finger.

The evaluation of sensation in third party liability situations requires a careful, thoughtful approach if abnormalities are found on examination. For example, if I am evaluating a patient with an upper extremity injury I may start by lightly stroking the skin on both shoulders and asking if this stroking feels the same on both sides. If a patient responds that the stroking feels the same at the shoulders, I follow with stroking of the lateral and medial upper arm, radial and ulnar forearm and all five digits. A normal patient will respond that the light stroking feels the same on both sides at each area of testing. If there has been, for example, a fracture of the wrist and I find decrease sensation of the radial digits, I will then look carefully for evidence of carpal tunnel syndrome.

An abnormal response to the quick light stroking sensation testing, which does not have an anatomic explanation, requires careful evaluation. Let's assume that the patient tells me that the stroking of the two shoulders feels different, I now wish to figure out if this has an anatomic explanation or not. I look for evidence of surgical or other scars which might explain an isolated area of decreased sensation of the shoulder. Not finding that, I ask does stroking of the lateral upper arm feel different. If I get a positive response, I continue down the arm as described above. If I continue to get responses of different light touch sensation from the patient, I move to the anterior chest, then upper the neck, then cheeks, then forehead, then down the body.

There are patients will give responses of altered light touch sensation for an entire arm or leg called stocking-glove hypesthesia. Others may give forequarter or hindquarter hypesthesia and occasionally hemi corpus hypesthesia. In the absence of other abnormalities, for example spinal cord dysfunction, these responses from a patient are not anatomic and are evidence of symptom magnification.

# CHAPTER TEN

# The brain – nerve – muscle – tendon - joint chain

This chapter covers the evaluation of brain, tendon, muscle, tendon, bone, joint functional chain. I wish to cover this as a separate system. Alterations in muscle/tendon function may occur from neurologic pathology, primary myopathology and abnormalities in the bone to tendon to muscle to tendon to skeletal attachment to joint abnormalities. In order for a motor unit, that is a muscle to function normally and move a joint, the pathway from brain volition, to spinal cord transmission, to motor neuron activation, to motor neuron axon conduction of the electrical impulse, to activation of the muscle, to contraction of the muscle, to active pulling on the tendons on both sides of the muscle, to moving a joint or joints all need to be intact. Failure of any link in this chain and the muscle movement will be absent or abnormal. I am presenting the examination of the brain-nerve-muscle-tendon-joint chain as a separate "system" for physical examination. An inability to move a specific joint normally may have a cause anywhere along the brain through joint chain.

Before testing for muscle function, it is necessary to ensure that the joints moved by the muscle in question move passively through a full range of motion. If the range of motion of a joint is limited, for example a frozen shoulder, then the evaluation of the muscle function must take the joint motion restriction into account.

If there is a question of generalized weakness or subtle weakness, examination for amyotrophic lateral sclerosis is indicated. Examine the tongue for fasciculations. Take off the patient's shirt. Sit and stare forward at the chest for at least 30 seconds waiting to see if your peripheral vision picks up occasional, subtle fasciculations. It is best to explain to your patient that you are going to stare straight ahead for 30 seconds looking for muscle flickers. Otherwise, your patient will think you are odder than you really are.

Quick Upper Extremity Muscle Exam

First, observation. Again, observation. Always, observation. Look for atrophy. Look for abnormal contour. Look for asymmetry of muscle size. Look for asymmetry of resting posture. Look for unusual movements.

Ask the patient to raise his arms above his head and to bend and straighten his elbows. This checks for full range of motion of the shoulders and elbows. Ask the patient to hold his arms out to the side and to push up against your downward push with your hands. This tests the deltoid muscles. Next, I ask the patient to push with his right hand against my pushing left hand. Simultaneously, I palpate the right scapula. This tests the right triceps and simultaneously the right serratus anterior muscle. If the right scapula wings out the right serratus anterior muscle is weak. Then I test the other side.

Next in my upper extremity examination, I ask the patient to bend his elbow and resist me as I try to straighten his elbow. This tests the biceps and brachioradialis muscles. If there is any question regarding weakness of the biceps, I shake hands with my patient with the elbow bent 90 degrees and then ask the patients to forcefully pronate and supinate the forearm against my resistance. The biceps muscle is the principal supinator of the forearm. Marked weakness of supination of the forearm suggests marked weakness or absence of biceps function. The brachioradialis muscle may provide strong flexion of the elbow against resistance in the absence of biceps function especially if the forearm is pronated.

Next, I ask the patient to grip tightly as I try to straighten the fingers. This tests the flexor digitorum profundus and flexor digitorum sublimis muscles grossly. If there is any question of weakness, I slow down and specifically test forced flexion against resistance for each distal interphalangeal joint and the interphalangeal joint of the thumb as well as forced flexion of the proximal interphalangeal joints. Flexion at the distal interphalangeal joints tests the flexor digitorum profundus. Flexion at the proximal interphalangeal joints while holding the other fingers in extension tests the flexor digitorum sublimis.

Next, I ask the patient extend his fingers and push up against resistance offered by my fingers. This tests the extensor digitorum communis muscle. I ask the patient to make a fist. While holding the fist, I asked the patient to extend the index finger and little finger against resistance. The index finger and the little finger have independent extensor muscles which will work even though the extensor digitorum communis muscle is prevented from working by the making of the fist.

Then, I ask the patient to spread his fingers as I gently try to push them together. This tests the first dorsal interosseus muscle and the abductor digiti quinti. Then I give the patient a sheet of paper to hold together with his straightened fingers. I then try to pull the paper away with my fingers holding the sheet of paper in the same way. This tests the volar interosseous muscles involved with the adducting fingers. I have the patient place his palms flat on a table and then try to elevate the thumb off of the table. This tests for function of the extensor pollicis longus muscle and tendon.

This quick survey of upper extremity muscles is not complete but is sufficiently thorough to pick up any generalized total body weakness, a brachial plexus injury, and palsies of the radial, median and ulnar nerves. This survey will also pick up injured muscles and lacerated or ruptured tendons. If any weakness is detected with this muscle strength survey, then more detailed testing is indicated.

**If there is a skin break from a laceration or even a small puncture wound, then the testing described above is necessary to look for an isolated nerve injury (two point discrimination testing) or a tendon laceration or lacerations.**

Many medical providers work in situations in which they are the first to evaluate injured patients. These medical providers may work in emergency rooms, 24 hour walk in clinics, offices of general practitioners, pediatricians and many other places. A knowledge of how to evaluate the upper extremity for tendon lacerations, spontaneous tendon ruptures and tendon avulsions is important. A knowledge of how to evaluate the upper extremity for nerve lacerations discussed in the previous chapter is important.

**If not specifically looked for in detail, many tendon and nerve lacerations will be missed. Missed nerve and tendon injuries are common, common, common.**

*Case Study:*
*A patient fell while skiing and injured his left shoulder. As part of my initial physical examination I ask him to lift his left arm over his head. He is unable to do this. If the patient is not asked to actively elevate his arm against gravity a massive tear of the rotator cuff may be missed. A patient may be unable to elevate the arm due to pain from a partial rotator cuff tear. If the patient is unable to elevate his arm actively he should be reexamined within a week after the pain has decreased to see if he is still unable to do so. If not specifically looked for, if not specifically examined for rotator cuff tears will be missed.*

*Is there harm if a massive rotator cuff tear is missed? Yes. After three weeks or so the contracted muscle scars and cannot be stretched out and surgical repair is more difficult and surgical results are not as good as they could be with early recognition. My patient returns after one week still unable to elevate his arm over his head. MRI shows a massive rotator cuff tear which requires surgical repair. From an anatomical point of view a rotator cuff tear is a tear at the muscle tendon junction or avulsion of tendon from its attachment.*

If there is lack of partial or full active motion at a joint. The next important step is to determine if there is passive motion. Lack of motion at a joint may be due to limited motion of the joint and/or lack of strength of the muscle.

*Case Study:*

*A patient came to my office complaining of right arm pain and weakness. He was holding on to the mast of a sailboat when he slipped and fell. In reflex he held on to the mast and hurt his arm as he fell. Immediate observation discloses bruising of the upper arm. This patient needs to be carefully evaluated for a ruptured biceps tendon. Observation of a relatively thin patient may disclose superior migration of the body of the biceps tendon. This will not be obvious in an obese patient.*

*My patient has full active flexion of the elbow against gravity. I ask the patient to flex the elbow against resistance with the forearm supinated. This is distinctly weak. If the biceps tendon is ruptured and elbow flexion is tested while the forearm is pronated, the brachioradialis may fool you into thinking the biceps tendon is intact. A major function of the biceps muscle is active supination of the forearm. I grasp my patient's hand like you are shaking hands and ask him to rotate against my supinating hand. Marked weakness. In a ruptured biceps tendon, supination will be weak. My patient chose surgical repair.*

*Case Study:*

*A patient came to my office complaining that he injured his left elbow while lifting weights. His main complaint is pain in the elbow. Initial observation sitting across from the patient is normal. His left arm rests in a normal posture. I elevate his arm so that the elbow points upward with the elbow flexed. I then ask my patient to straighten his elbow against gravity. He is unable to do this. I palpate deeply just proximal to the olecranon and sense a deep defect at the site of the triceps attachment. X-rays are negative for fracture. This patient has a ruptured triceps tendon.*

*You can test elbow extension against gravity by having the patient elevate his elbow up toward the ceiling and rest his hand on his head. Then ask him to straighten his elbow. Alternatively, have the patient lie on his side with the affected elbow up and the elbow bent. Ask the patient to straighten his elbow. Ruptured triceps tendons are not common but may be missed.*

*Case Study:*
*A patient comes to my office complaining of a weak thumb. Initial observation with the patient sitting with his arms in his lap is normal. I ask the patient to hold his hands in the air. Observation now shows the thumb tends to hang down a little more than the other side. I ask my patient to place his hand flat on a table top palm down. Then, while leaving the hand flat on the table I ask the patient to elevate his thumb up off of the table toward the ceiling. He cannot do it. This patient has a spontaneous rupture of the extensor pollicis longus tendon. This tendon makes a sharp angle turn as it travels from the forearm to the dorsum of the thumb. This sharp angle may contribute to the cause of the occasional spontaneous rupture. This test should be used for any laceration of the dorsum of the hand or wrist to look for a laceration of this tendon. Laceration of the extensor policies longus tendon is another diagnosis frequently missed. Why missed? Missed due to a failure to perform this specific test for the integrity of the extensor policies longus tendon.*

*Case Study:*
*A patient with a history of rheumatoid arthritis was referred with the complaint of thumb weakness. A careful and detailed examination showed absence of function of the flexor of the interphalangeal joint of the thumb, the flexor polli-*

*cis longus. The patient was not aware that this was the cause of her complaint of weakness. This was not diagnosed by the referring physician, rheumatologist. This was a spontaneous rupture of the flexor policies longus tendon and required surgery to clean out inflamed synovial tissue, trim down a bone spur and perform a tendon transfer taking the flexor digitorum sublimis to the ring finger and attaching it to the distal end of the ruptured thumb flexor tendon.*

*Case Study:*

*A patient comes to my office complaining of a stiff, sprained right ring finger which is not getting better. He was playing tackle football and sprained his finger while grabbing onto an opposing player's shirt. He was seen in an emergency room one month previously by an emergency room physician. He was told that he had a sprained finger and the finger was splinted in a straight position. This patient was followed up by his general practitioner who continued the splinting.*

*Careful observation in my office shows that the right ring finger's position of rest is more extended than the other fingers. On careful palpation, there is swelling and tenderness volar to the proximal phalanx of the right ring finger. Careful detailed muscle/tendon testing discloses absence of active flexion of the distal phalangeal joint of the right ring finger.*

*This is a "rugger jersey injury." Make a fist with your four fingers. While holding a tight fist, sequentially try to passively extend each finger. You will find that the index, middle and little finger extend much further than the ring finger. The distal phalanx of the ring finger remains more flexed than the distal phalanges of the other fingers, if the other fingers remain in a tight fist. If the isolated ring finger is holding on to an object, a shirt for example, while that object is pulled forcefully away, the extensor force on the distal phalanx may be sufficient to avulse the flexor digitorum profundus (with or without fracture) from the distal phalanx. This injury is frequently missed in the initial evaluation of "sprained ring fingers." By frequently missed, I mean, frequently missed. Delay in treatment may significantly harm the final result of treatment. I repeat, this injury is frequently missed due to failure to test for active flexion of the distal phalanx of the ring finger. All "sprained fingers" should be tested for tendon function.*

Why have I inserted so many case studies of various tendon ruptures? Tendon ruptures and tendon lacerations are common enough, that if you work in a medical environment in which you evaluate and treat "sprained fingers" and other joints, you will miss them unless you perform a careful and thorough evaluation on each and every patient. Tendon ruptures often present with minor complaints of pain. The lack of serious pain complaint may lull you into an incomplete physical examination.

Quick Lower Extremity Muscle/Tendon Exam

The quick lower extremity muscle exam may be performed with the patient sitting or lying supine. Ask the patient to flex her hip to 90 degrees and then hold against firm pressure with your hand trying to extend the hip joint. This tests the iliopsoas muscle.

*Case Study:*
*I was called to perform an orthopedic consultation on an inpatient. The patient was in her mid 30s and noted the spontaneous onset of right hip pain and inability to walk. The patient had already been evaluated by an internist, a physiatrist and a neurologist with no clear diagnosis. My detailed muscle examination disclosed marked weakness of the right hip flexor, that is marked weakness of the right iliopsoas muscle. The rest of the muscle testing was normal in detail. Sensation was intact to light touch sensation for the entire right lower extremity.*

*With a nurse as chaperone, I examined the skin around the proximal hip and perineal area. There was a linear vesicular rash present on the proximal, anterior, medial thigh. This patient's pain and weakness were caused by shingles of the proximal right leg. Unusual case. Only one I ever saw of shingles of the leg. Only case I ever saw of isolated weakness of the iliopsoas muscle.*

*I keep commenting on the need for thoughtful and thorough observation. I keep commenting on the need for careful, thoughtful and thorough physical examinations. The three previous physicians were good, competent doctors. The three previous physicians failed to examine the skin around the hip area as part of their hip examination. Why? Possibly due to reticence to expose the upper thigh and perineal area of a woman for their physical examinations. Possibly due to failure to follow a protocol which involves a "complete" hip examination including evaluation of the skin.*

Ask the patient to straighten her knee and then hold the knee straight against firm pressure with your hand. This tests the quadriceps muscle. The start of this test should have the patient simply holding his knee straight against gravity. If you start your quadriceps muscle test with straightening the leg against gravity, you will automatically pick up an unexpected rupture of the quadriceps tendon. You may not think this injury can be missed. I have seen missed quadriceps ruptures three times in my career. Surprisingly, patients are sometimes able to walk with a ruptured quadriceps muscle by maximally straightening their knee during stance phase. Yes, a patient may come to your office walking and still have a ruptured quadriceps muscle.

*Case Study:*
*A 46 year old man was referred to my office for treatment of a sprained knee. He walked into my office without apparent difficulty. I first saw him sitting on the examination table with the knees flexed. I took the medical history with him sitting on the examination table. I asked the patient to straighten his knee. Since he was sitting on the exam table I was asking him to extend his knee against gravity. He was unable to do it. Deep palpation disclosed a defect in the quadriceps tendon just superior to the patella. A clear case of ruptured quadriceps tendon. Note: Rarely patients will rupture both quadriceps tendons at the same time.*

Inability to straighten the knee against gravity can also be caused by a patellar fracture and rupture of the patellar tendon. With rupture of the patellar tendon the patellar will often ride up proximally.

If the patient extends his knee against gravity, then have him extend the knee against resistance. Have the patient flex his knee and hold against a firm pull trying to straighten the knee. This tests the hamstring muscles. In the case of a hamstring muscle strain or avulsion of the hamstring origin from the pelvis, this will be painful. Have the patient dorsiflex the ankle against resistance. This tests the tibialis anterior muscle. Be aware that the toe extensors also have some ankle dorsiflexion activity.

Have the patient plantarflex the ankle against resistance. This tests the gastrocnemius and soleus muscles. Be aware that the toe flexors may provide active plantar flexion of the ankle in the presence of a ruptured Achilles tendon. You may be fooled into thinking the Achilles tendon is intact due to the active plantar flexion of the ankle by the toe flexors.

*Case Study:*
*A 36 year old man comes to my office complaining of a right ankle sprain. He was playing rugby. He turned and pushed off with his right foot. He felt immediate pain, like an opposing player had kicked him in the back of his ankle. He fell down with pain in his ankle. On examination he demonstrates active plantar flexion of his right ankle.*

*I ask the patient to kneel on the exam table facing the wall. I gently squeeze both calves sequentially. On the left side the ankle passively plantar flexes when the left calf is squeezed. On the right side squeezing the calf results in no motion of the right ankle. This is the Thompson test for evaluating the possibility of a ruptured Achilles tendon. In this case the Thompson test was positive for a ruptured Achilles tendon on the right. Deep palpation disclosed a palpable defect just proximal to the posterior calcaneus. In Achilles tendon ruptures which are more proximal, a palpable defect may not be obvious. Failure to appreciate a palpable defect in the distal Achilles tendon does not rule out a ruptured Achilles tendon.*

*The Thompson test may also be performed with a patient lying prone. I liked the kneeling method. I had my patients turn and look over their shoulders, My patients could see the difference in the two sides and recognized clearly that the Achilles tendon was ruptured.*

*The key point of this case study is the fact that in patients with a rupture of the Achilles tendon, testing for active flexion of the ankle may demonstrate that some active flexion of the ankle from the action of the toe flexors. This may fool you into thinking the Achilles tendon is intact. The thorough and careful way to evaluate the possibility of a ruptured Achilles tendon is to perform the Thompson test. In looking up the Thompson test, I see that it is also called the Simmond's test. I know it by the Thompson test name. This test needs to be done for any leg or ankle injury which is not an obvious displaced fracture. I have seen this injury missed on occasion. Patients may walk on a rupture Achilles tendon. The fact that a patient walks in to your office does not rule out this diagnosis.*

Ruptured Achilles tendons may not be particularly painful. As a general rule, partial ligament tears are more painful than complete tears. In a complete tendon avulsion or ligament tear, motion does not put a strain on the injured structures. In a partial tear, any motion pulls on the injured structure causing pain.

Continuing the muscle exam of the ankle. Forced inversion of the ankle against resistance tests the posterior tibial muscle. Forced eversion of the ankle against resistance tests the peroneal muscles. Isolated weakness of ankle eversion may be a sign of a peroneal nerve palsy. While testing forced eversion of the ankle, close observation of the lateral malleolus will pick up occasional subluxation of the peroneal tendons. Forced dorsiflexion of the big toe tests the extensor hallucis longus muscle.

Testing the muscles of the lower extremity may fail to disclose subtle weakness because the leg muscles are much stronger than the resistance provided by the upper extremity muscles of the examining medical provider. If there is a question regarding subtle weakness of the lower extremity muscles, ask the patient to perform ten toe rises with each leg while supporting himself. This tests the gastrocnemius and soleus muscles. Ask the patient to perform heel walking. This tests the tibialis anterior muscles. Ask the patient to rise up from a squatting position. Failure to perform any of these tests may indicate subtle muscle weakness.

*Case Study*

*I am going through my list of preoperative medical histories and physical exams at Children's Hospital in Boston, as a beginning orthopedic resident. One of the patients on my list is a male teenager with scoliosis scheduled for reconstructive surgery the next morning. I enter the hospital room and find him lying down on the hospital bed. After taking his history, I move on to the part of the physical examination I can do with the patient supine. This part of the exam is normal. I then ask the patient to stand up so that I can examine his back in a standing position.*

*He gets up quickly and stands up. Something about the way he sits up triggers my observational antennae. He seems to use his arms to elevate himself more than I think is normal. The apparent unusual use of his arms is subtle. I am not sure. Something seems a little off. Once again, I emphasize the importance of thoughtful and thorough observation. I ask this patient to lie down again and sit up without using his arms. He replies, "I can't." He has never complained about this to anyone.*

*Further evaluation documented late onset muscular dystrophy. This was missed by his pediatrician. This was missed by the professor of pediatric orthopedic surgery at Children's Hospital in Boston, who had seen him before his scheduled surgery. In retrospect, the fact that his scoliosis was single curve in a male teen-*

*ager should have been an indication to search for other causes of his scoliosis. Most scoliosis patients have double curves on x-ray. Neither the pediatrician nor the full professor of pediatric orthopedic surgery "observed" the fact that the single scoliosis curve was a "statistical outlier" deserving further evaluation.*

*I think that asking a patient to perform a sit up without using arms or hands is a potentially useful muscle test for the early detection of patients with muscle dystrophies. It was the key physical examination finding in this patient which allowed me, an early first year orthopedic resident, to recognize that this patient had muscle weakness requiring further evaluation.*

*Case Study:*
*An 18 year old male comes to my office complaining of bilateral shoulder pain. He has no other complaints. This is an unusual complaint in a patient this age. A complaint of bilateral shoulder pain in an 18 year old is sufficiently unusual that already my antennae are quivering looking for a statistical outlier diagnosis. To start my upper extremity physical exam, I ask the patient to elevate his arms over his head. As mentioned before, this is my quick examination start which looks for range of motion of the shoulders and deltoid muscle function. He raises his arms over his head quickly. Something about the way he elevates his arms concerns me. He seems to throw his arms up, not unlike someone lifting more weight than they should, who throws the weight up quickly with their arm. Again, my emphasis on the need for thoughtful and careful observation. I am not sure. But, I have a sense that he seems to throw his arms up faster than normal.*

*I ask him to raise his arms up slowly. He replies, "I can't." I take off his shirt. I see marked atrophy of the proximal shoulder girdle on both sides. EMGs confirm fascio scapular humeral dystrophy. His pediatrician, who referred this patient, missed the diagnosis.*

Part of a muscle exam may include the measurement of the circumferences of extremities as a way to look for and document asymmetry in muscle size. Asymmetry of the size and circumference of the arms and legs may have causes other than primary nerve or muscle dysfunction. For the upper arm measure the maximum circumference of the relaxed biceps muscle. For the forearm five inches above the radial styloid is one often used level for measuring forearm circumference. For the thigh five inches above the medial knee joint line is often used. For the calf the maximum circumference of the gastrocnemius soleus muscle complex.

There are numerous provocative tests used in evaluating patients. A cardiac stress test is, in essence, a provocative test looking for ischemic EKG changes when the heart is stressed. In a sense, reflex testing and Tinel's sign testing are provocative tests. In orthopedic evaluations, provocative tests are often used to examine for possible ligament instability, joint instability, tendon subluxation and abnormal pain or numbness or tingling with certain maneuvers. These tests will be covered in the sections covering the specific anatomic areas.

# CHAPTER ELEVEN

# The need for specific protocols in conducting each and every physical examination

Why am I continuing to emphasize the need to develop specific, detailed, complete protocols for performing each and every physical examination you perform? If you fail to utilize a specific, detailed complete protocol each and every time you examine a patient, you increase your chances of missing abnormalities. If you fail to utilize a specific protocol each and every time, you increase your chances of missing important diagnoses. Similarly, when treating patients, there are often specific treatment protocols which need to be followed. This is not unlike pilots utilizing a specific pre-flight check before each and every flight. Am I overstating the case? Here are some case studies in which the utilization of protocols was important.

*Case Study:*

*I am working in a suburban emergency room when an ambulance rolls in with an unconscious patient. The immediate quick observation part of the physical exam shows a middle aged man, unconscious with his arms in rigid decerebrate posturing. The arms and legs are rigidly extended and the arms are internally rotated. I saw this patient in the early 1970s before the availability of emergency CT or MRI scans. This was clearly a severe stroke with a poor prognosis. There was really nothing to do. Was there?*

*And. Yet! And. Yet! And. Yet!*

*Fortunately, and I do mean fortunately, I remembered the <u>unconscious proto-</u><u>col</u>. I drew a blood sugar, sent it to the lab and gave the patient an ampule of D50W, a concentrated sugar solution. I was following the unconscious protocol robotically with no expectation of this being helpful. Twenty seconds later, the patient woke up and was neurologically normal. His blood sugar came back 46.*

*I have told this story of an unusual presentation of insulin shock to numerous internists and emergency room physicians. None have seen this. Perhaps this patient had some brain abnormality which caused him to go into decerebrate posturing when severely hypoglycemic. I don't know. I present this case as a dramatic, teaching lesson on the importance of following examination and treatment protocols.*

*Case Study:*

*I am working in a suburban emergency room. A man calls the emergency room and asks to speak to the doctor on call. He speaks normally evidencing no distress. He tells me that he fell down the basement stairs and hurt his neck. I tell him to come in to the emergency room for evaluation and treatment. Perhaps half an hour later a nurse tells me that the patient, who called on the phone, is on a stretcher in the hallway. I walk over to see him. He is lying on the stretcher supine in no distress. Following their standard protocol, the emergency medical technicians who brought him in to the emergency room by ambulance, placed a firm neck collar around his neck. Do I remove his collar in order to examine his neck?*

*I take his medical history. I ask for details regarding his fall down the stairs and his mechanism of injury. He now tells me that he fell down a full flight of stairs backwards, hitting his head. He tells me that when he called me, he was lying upside down on the stairs with his head at an angle against the wall at the bottom of the stairs.*

*With this history I follow the neck injury protocol (for that time) and take wide adhesive tape and tape from one side of the stretcher to his forehead to the other side of the stretcher. This, with the firm collar in place, completely immobilizes his neck. I send him to x-ray for a lateral cervical spine view only with the patient immobilized. This and then other views show an unstable cervical spine fracture at serious risk of displacing and damaging his spinal cord. I call in a spine surgeon to oversee further care.*

*The protocol of protecting the neck until the question of possible unstable cervical spine fracture is answered prevented any possible damage to the spinal cord. Here the protocol was immediate and total protection of the neck while proceeding to evaluate the patient.*

*Case Study:*
*This case was told to me by a friend. I present this case more for human interest and humor than for its teaching value. He was working in the emergency room of a large intercity hospital. A patient walked up to the triage nurse's desk complaining of back pain. The patient stated that he had been stabbed in the back. He did not appear to be in distress. The triage nurse asked him to take a seat and told him he would be called back when his turn came. Approximately half an hour later my friend walked out in to the waiting room to talk to another patient's family. My friend happened to glance around the waiting room. He*

noticed the patient I just mentioned above. He was sitting patiently in a chair with a knife sticking out of his back.

The patient had neglected to tell the triage nurse that the knife was still in his back. The triage nurse had not asked the patient to turn around in order to look at his back or the wound as part of the triaging of this patient. Perhaps if the triage nurse had watched the patient as he turned around to walk to a chair he would have seen the knife. I suppose it is safe to say that the triage nurse did not take a sufficiently detailed history nor did he perform a sufficiently detailed triage physical examination.

**My lesson here is simple. Your protocol for examination of each part of the body should be sufficiently thorough and complete that you will pick up subtle and unusual abnormalities. If you fail to develop protocols for your physical examination that are sufficiently thorough, you will miss diagnoses in your career. If you fail to develop the habit of carefully observation you will miss diagnoses in your career. If you allow yourself to get lazy and skimp on your physical examinations you will miss diagnoses in your career.**

# CHAPTER TWELVE:
# Physical Examination of The Cardiovascular System

---

# Cardiovasculi Omnia est divisa partes tres

---

I am going to continue my discussion of the physical examination partly by physiologic system and partly by anatomic part of the body. There is no special reason for the order I have chosen.

For simplicity and organization, I divide the physical examination of the cardiovascular system into three parts as Julius Caesar divided Gaul into three parts: namely, the heart sounds, the heartbeat rhythm (ie. pulse rhythm) and the peripheral vascular system.

The first part of the cardiovascular exam involves general observation. Always observation. Is there cyanosis? Is there obvious dyspnea? Is the patient breathing rapidly? Are the ankles swollen?

*Case Study:*

*A 68 year old woman is referred to my office by the emergency room with a fractured wrist. As I sit across from her and begin to talk to her I note bilateral swollen ankles. Before asking about her wrist and possible numbness and tingling, I ask if she is seeing an internist or cardiologist. Yes, she is seeing a cardiologist. Yes, she has been told she has a "weak" heart. She hasn't seen her cardiologist for four months. After completing my history and physical examination, I call the cardiologist. Four months ago, her congestive heart failure was under control.*

*The swollen ankles are a clear sign she is retaining fluid and that her congestive heart failure is not under control. She has 4+ pitting edema of her ankles extending up to her proximal tibias. She is clearly not a surgical candidate for treatment of her wrist fracture. I decide on nonoperative treatment and arrange to have the patient go directly to the cardiologist's office.*

*This patient came to my office for treatment of her wrist fracture. Observation of her ankles led to another diagnosis, uncontrolled congestive heart failure. Observation of her ankles led to my decision to avoid surgical treatment of her wrist fracture. Observation of her ankles led me to have her see her cardiologist the same day I saw her.*

The Heart Sounds

The first heart sound, called S1 is made by the closing of the tricuspid valve and the mitral valve. These are the valves between the right atrium and right ventricle and between the left atrium and left ventricle. As the ventricles contract, the pressure in the ventricles becomes greater than the pressure in the atria and the valves "snap" shut. The two valves snap shut almost simultaneously, thus S1 sounds like only one sound and not two.

The second heart sound called S2 comes from the closing of the pulmonary and aortic valves. This occurs when the ventricle relaxes and the pressure in the pulmonary artery and in the aorta becomes greater than the pressure in the relaxing ventricles. The sound of S2 sounds split because the greater pressure in the aorta causes the aortic valve to snap shut (A2) a little before the pulmonary valve snaps shut (P2).

Whoosh sounds between the sounds of S1 and S2, if heard, are likely due to some abnormal flow of blood. These abnormal sounds are called murmurs and are graded one to four. One is barely perceptible and four can be heard across a room. The grading of murmurs is highly subjective and clearly changes as the auscultator ages and his hearing decreases. Note: my internists and cardiologists have not reacted well to my joking suggestions that their grading of murmurs is changing as they age.

Murmurs which occur after the first heart sound are called systolic murmurs. If present may indicate stenosis of the aortic valve or incompetence of the mitral valve among other causes. Incompetence of the mitral valve may occur in rheumatic heart disease, from rupture of the chordae tendineae or cardiac ischemia. Subacute bacterial endocarditis may also lead to incompetence of the heart valves.

Murmurs which occur after the second heart sound are called diastolic murmurs. If present may indicate mitral valve stenosis or aortic valve incompetence among other causes.

When auscultating to the heart it is important to specifically listen for rubs. This may indicate pericarditis from spontaneous inflammation or from ischemia.

The stethoscope is moved from the upper left anterior chest gradually down and around to the lower anterior lateral chest in order to listen to the heart from different locations. The upper anterior chest will hear the right side of the heart better. The lower left side of the chest is closer to the left ventricle and will hear that side of the heart better. Using the flat side of the stethoscope and the bell side expands your ability to distinguish higher and lower pitch sounds.

*Case Study:*

*My first day of our Introduction to the Clinic rotation. I arrive at a room at the Massachusetts General Hospital. The teacher hands me a piece of paper with a patient's name, ward and bed number. My patient is in a corner bed of a 30 patient ward with the curtains drawn around him. I walk in. The patient is unconscious. So, no history can be taken. Learning to take a medical history will have to wait for another day. I take out my stethoscope in order to auscultate the heart and place the stethoscope over the anterior left chest. No heartbeat! I check. The patient is alive and breathing. I listen over the anterior left chest. Still no heartbeat. I hold the stethoscope over my heart to ascertain if it is working. It is.*

*I give up on trying to listen to the heart. I move on to examining the lungs. When I put the stethoscope over the right anterior chest I hear the heart beat loud and clear. I then notice that the trachea is deviated to the right. This patient has end stage lung cancer with a collapsed right lung. The entire mediastinum including the heart has shifted to the right.*

Heartbeat Rhythm

The heartbeat rhythm may be detected from any location where a pulse is detected or from listening to the heart. Obviously, if abnormalities are detected work up immediately moves on to an EKG or ECG (electrocardiogram).

There are basically three types of heart beat rhythms. Regular rhythm which is the typical lub dub, lub dub, lub dub, lub dub, etc. If the heart rate, i.e. number of beats per minute, is typical for age, then this is a normal sinus rhythm. Competitive athletes may have an unusually low heart rate which is normal, given their history of athletic training. A very slow regular heart rhythm, under 45, may be a sign of heart block. In heart block the electrical signals from the left atrium are blocked and do not reach the left ventricle. The ventricles may then develop a slow rhythm of their own.

If there is a regular rhythm which is much faster than normal this indicates other electrical abnormalities. Regular heart rates of 100 to 130 may be due to stress, infection and left atrial abnormalities. Regular heart rates of 130 t0 150 beats per minutes may be called paroxysmal atrial tachycardia.

There are heartbeat rhythms which are irregular, but irregular in a regular or periodic fashion. These are called regular irregular rhythms. I do so love medical terminology. If there are extra atrial or ventricular beats which occur on a regular, periodic basis, this may cause a regular irregular rhythm. Thus, a rhythm which goes lub dub, short pause, lub dub, long pause, lub dub short pause, lub dub long pause, etc. is such a heartbeat rhythm.

Lastly, there is the irregular, irregular rhythm. This is often seen with atrial fibrillation. In this problem the left atrium is like a wriggling mass of worms and does not beat regularly. The more or less random electrical firings of the atrial cells leak into the ventricle in a random unpredictable fashion. Thus, the electrical signals to the left ventricle arrive randomly and the heartbeat rhythm is correspondingly random. It may be difficult to be sure what you are feeling if you are taking a peripheral pulse. This diagnosis is important to detect early because of risk of stroke from blood clots which form on the inner cardiac wall.

Ventricular tachycardia is a rapid heart rate. The electrical impulses arise in the ventricles. In many cases this is a potentially serious and life threatening situation particularly if the heartrate is fast.

Peripheral Pulses

Temporal artery pulse

There are superficial arteries at locations which allow for the detection of pulses and or bruits at many parts of the body. Starting from the top: Temporal arteritis or giant cell arteritis may present with headaches and/or scalp tenderness and /or jaw pain and/or vision problems. If undiagnosed and untreated the risk of vision loss increases. Loss of the temporal artery pulse may indicate this diagnosis. Certainly, asymmetry in the temporal artery pulses should be a concern. Feeling for the temporal artery pulse should be part of every headache, head pain and vision change physical examination.

Carotid Pulse

The carotid artery pulse is easily felt by gently palpating deep between the trachea and the sternocleidomastoid muscle. In the middle age to older population palpation should specifically felt looking for asymmetry. The carotids should also be auscultated specifically listening for bruits. Carotid artery stenosis is a serious risk factor for stroke. Any bruits detected should undergo further evaluation.

Thoracic Outlet

There is no specific "pulse" available for physical examination in the thoracic outlet area. There is a syndrome called the thoracic outlet syndrome. Occasionally medical terminology makes a little sense. Symptoms occur when there is compression of blood vessels or nerves as they cross the thoracic outlet. Common causes include anatomical defects such as an extra rib and physical trauma either acute or repetitive. Often there is no clear cause other than the outlet is narrower than normal.

Adson's test is often used to examine for thoracic outlet syndrome. My memory, from reading Adson's original paper years ago is that he actually described more than one test for thoracic outlet syndrome. If someone tells you that they performed an Adson test on a patient, there is room for confusion, since clinicians perform this test differently. I was taught to feel for a patient's radial pulse (see below) with the patient's arm that his/her side. Then, I bring the arm of the examined side up into a shoulder abducted position. I also rotate the patient's head to the opposite side and lateral bend the patient's head away from the abducted arm. Some clinicians have the patients hold their breath.

You, the clinician, are looking for loss of radial pulse and recreation of the patient's complaints of arm numbness, tingling or pain. Loss of radial pulse during the Adson's test occurs often, has a high false positive rate and taken alone is not a significant finding.

Thoracic outlet syndrome is rare. The diagnosis is difficult. The Adson test is probably of marginal value. To make this diagnosis the clinical has to be looking for it. Performing the Adson test during arteriography is more definitive. There are rare patients with clear and distinctive responses to the Adson test as I have described. The test should be performed as part of any work up of arm pain or arm numbness or tingling of unclear etiology.

Thoracic outlet syndrome may be symptomatic more from nerve pressure than from vascular pressure. This seemed as good a place to discuss it as anywhere.

Brachial Artery Pulse

This is felt medially in the distal part of the upper arm. It is important only if there is serious concern regarding blood supply to the upper arm. When I was in training the brachial artery was a frequent site we used for obtaining arterial blood for study.

Wrist Pulses

The radial pulse is probably the most frequently used pulse for checking heart rate and heart beat rhythm. It is at the volar radial wrist between the radial styloid and the flexor carpi radialis tendon. The ulnar pulse is often hard to feel. Inability to feel the ulnar pulse does not always indicate a specific problem.

Allen's Test

The Allen's test allows for the physical examination of the patency of arteries when there are two arteries providing blood supply to a part of the anatomy. This test is used mostly at the wrist and the base of the fingers.

To perform the Allen's test, gently compress the radial and ulnar arteries at the wrist with each of your thumbs. Then have the patient open and close his fist a few times to squeeze blood out of the hand. Then have the patient hold his hand with the fingers gently extended. Then, release one of the arteries and observe the extent of blood flow into the hand. Then, repeat the sequence but release the other artery and again observe the return of blood flow to the hand after release.

A normal result is immediate restoration of blood flow to the entire hand after release of each artery. Normally, there are sufficient cross connections of circulation for this to occur. When might you find abnormalities with the Allen's Test at the wrist? Peripheral arterial disease, peripheral emboli lodging in the upper extremity and Buerger's disease (thromboangiitis obliterans) are a few. A patient who had a radial artery line in an intensive care unit might have thrombosis of the radial artery. Ulnar artery thrombosis at the wrist is probably more common than recognized. One cause is the repetitive use of heel of the hand as a hammer, called hypothenar hammer syndrome.

For most patient's the radial and ulnar arteries are the predominant source of blood supply to the hand. Occasional patients have a persistent median artery which is present in the fetus and usually disappears. In those patients in whom it persists it is a continuation of the anterior interosseous artery. There may be a false negative Allen's test result in this anatomic abnormality situation.

Fingers

There is no specific finger pulse available for exam. Occasional patients will have blackening or crusting of the tip of one or more fingers. This may be necrosis of the skin at the tips of the fingers from severe peripheral arterial disease of the upper extremity. The Allen's test of the fingers involves massaging the blood out of the fingers from distal to proximal and immediately pressing gently on the volar lateral aspect of both sides of the finger which you are examining. This pressure compresses both digital arteries. Wait a few moments to ensure that the finger remains blanched. Then release the digital artery of one side and observe the finger for immediate return of blood flow. Repeat the procedure and release the digital artery on the other side. This will give information regarding the patency of the two digital arteries in the examined finger.

Abdominal Aorta

A normal abdominal aorta will not be palpable. A normal abdominal aorta will not make a sound capable of being heard by stethoscope. The only way you will detect an abdominal aortic aneurysm is by deep palpation during which you feel a pulsatile mass or by auscultation during which you hear a bruit. A pulsatile mass in the central abdomen may be a large aortic aneurysm and warrants immediate investigation. If this pulsatile mass is associated with complaints of severe back pain this is an emergency. This may be an actively dissecting abdominal aortic aneurysm. A bruit heard in the abdomen may indicate either severe stenosis of the abdominal aorta or an abdominal aortic aneurysm.

Inguinal Pulses and the Popliteal Pulses

The inguinal pulses are useful for puncture entry for arteriography. I have not found them particularly useful in physical examination. If there is significant decrease in arterial flow to the lower extremity this becomes obvious when examining lower pulses, capillary refill of the toes, hair growth of the toes and lower legs, skin discoloration of the lower legs and/or necrosis of the toes.

Ankle and Foot Pulses

The dorsalis pedis pulse and the posterior tibial pulse are useful in evaluating arterial blood supply to the lower leg. Evaluating these pulses requires a soft, deft palpation and time to feel for the pulse. The use of a Doppler machine increases the sensitivity of evaluating these pulses.

My quick evaluation of blood supply to the lower leg and foot involves looking for hair growth on the toes. Even women who shave their legs often leave hair on the toes. If there is hair growth on the toes, then there is sufficient blood supply to the feet. Evaluating blood supply to the lower legs and feet is important in every yearly physical examination. It is also important in evaluating any patient with claudication symptoms. Examining the blood to the legs and feet is also critical as a preoperative evaluation before any surgery to the legs or feet.

I have seen numerous patients who have symptoms from both vascular insufficiency and lumbar spinal stenosis. As I stated earlier, always look for more than one diagnosis. Patients with claudication may have both lumbar spinal stenosis and atherosclerotic peripheral vascular disease. I repeat, adequate blood supply to the feet and lower extremity should be verified before planning or performing any lower extremity surgery.

Diabetics should be told to examine their feet every day looking for black area or ulcers which are evidence of necrosis. Shoes and socks should be removed and the feet examined at every, that is, every visit with a medical provider, regardless of specialty.

Venous System

The most common abnormalities of the venous system are varicose veins of the legs. Varicosities will not be evident if you only examine a patient supine lying in bed. With a patient standing bulging varicose veins may be visually observed. They may be palpated by digital compression and then watching the filling of the varicosity on release of the pressure. The area of the skin over the varicosity may feel warmer than expected. In chronic cases the skin discolors and ulcers may form. Rare cases of upper extremity venous thrombosis may present with skin discoloration.

Lymphatics

Blockage of lymph flow may occur for congenital reasons or following radiation. The physical findings may include soft tissue swelling and a woody type of edema. There will often be pitting edema. In pitting edema, the examiner pushes gently in on the soft tissue. On release of the pressure the indentation persists and only slowly disappears. This is often unilateral.

In congestive heart failure edema of the feet, ankles and lower legs will be equal bilaterally unless there is some co-existing unilateral problem.

Part of any yearly physical examination and for many other examinations palpation for lymphadenopathy should be performed. The most common locations for palpating for lymphadenopathy are the neck, the axillae and the groin.

# CHAPTER THIRTEEN:

# Physical Examination of the Chest and Pulmonary System

Again, observation. Is the patient sitting comfortably or in distress? What is his breathing rate? What is her skin color? What is the chest shape and size? Some patients with emphysema develop a slight barrel chest. Patients with relatively short stature and large barrel chests may come from populations which have adapted to high altitude environments such as the altiplano in Bolivia and Peru.

Palpation of the chest wall is indicated for complaints of chest wall pain following injury or if the pain develops spontaneously. Palpation may find tenderness of a rib or multiple ribs indicating possible rib fractures from injury or pathologic reasons. Patients with costochondritis may be tender to precise palpation at the costochondral junctions. This often occurs in the upper ribs.

From a straightforward point of view the physical examination of the pulmonary system seems simple. You have the left and right lung. Each has an upper, middle and lower lobe. As you listen to the lungs, i.e. auscultate the lungs, you move the stethoscope and listen to the front and back of the three lobes of each lung. Depending on your concerns you also auscultate around the sides of the chest wall.

The trick, if you will, is to listen carefully and not as a rote, boring exercise. You listen for rhonchi which are large tube sounds, rales which are small airway sounds and rubs. You also listen for what you don't hear. That is, is there a part of the lung with decreased breathing sounds? Rubs, in particular, may be faint. You have to listen for them and consciously ask yourself if you are hearing them. If you don't listen for them specifically, you will probably miss them. Percussion of the lower portions of each lung may indicate a pleural effusion if there is dullness inferiorly.

# CHAPTER FOURTEEN:
# The Physical Examination of the Breast

Before covering the technique of breast examination, let me ask a question. When should you examine a patient's breasts? Francis D. Moore, my chief of surgery at the Peter Bent Brigham hospital in the early 1970s insisted that every, and he meant every, physical examination of a woman should include a breast examination looking to pick up possible early cancers. Regardless of the reason for the physical exam. I repeat: regardless of the reason for the physical examination. If Dr. Moore found a record of a physical examination in which you failed to perform a breast exam, you got into trouble.

In today's world, patients will question a doctor performing a breast exam unless there is a specific, obvious reason for the breast exam. If I am performing a preoperative physical examination for an orthopedic problem, I ask female patients forty years old or older if they are getting regular mammograms. If they say yes, I move on with my history. If they say no, I ask if they want a cancer screening breast exam and then follow their wishes.

The first part of the breast examination, as always, involves observation. You look for asymmetry, skin changes, obvious masses and nipple discharge. In advanced, untreated breast cancer, the skin will look thickened and almost leather-like. This is called peau de orange or skin of the orange. I saw this once during my training in Boston. It is rare in the United States today.

You examine the breast with the patient lying supine and then sitting up. You palpate with your fingertips with light, medium and deep pressure. You sequentially exam the four quadrants of each breast feeling for consistency, tenderness and nodules. If you feel nodules you examine further for location, size, mobility and shape. You examine from the clavicle to the inframammary fold and from the sternum to the posterior axillary line. You examine for any asymmetry which might indicate a cancer.

# CHAPTER FIFTEEN:

# Physical Examination of the Abdomen

With my patient lying supine on the exam table I often will place my hand gently on the abdomen while talking with the patient. I wish to evaluate the patient's reaction to my gentle touching and to look for unexpected tenderness. Then I have the patient flex the hips and knees and place his feet on the table. This relaxes the abdominal muscles.

I press gently on the center of the abdomen looking for grimacing or other evidence that this maneuver is causing pain. If there is no evidence of pain I push a little deeper, again looking for evidence of pain. If there is no tenderness I push deeply feeling for an abdominal aortic aneurysm. If this is all normal, I move on to my structured exam. If there is evidence of pain with my palpation, I gently push deeper and then suddenly remove my hand. This maneuver "shakes" the abdominal contents. If this causes increased pain this is rebound tenderness. If there is tenderness I gently press the center and the four quadrants of the abdomen trying to find a location of greater tenderness.

Patients with peritonitis will be painful all over the abdomen and have marked rebound tenderness. Patients with early appendicitis may have tenderness limited to the right lower quadrant. Patients with diverticulitis may have left lower quadrant tenderness. Patients with hepatitis and other liver pathology may have right upper quadrant tenderness. Patients with an enlarged spleen or injured spleen may have left upper quadrant tenderness. This list is obviously limited. I am not writing a textbook on abdominal pathophysiology.

If I have not located a specific area of tenderness I move on. I percuss and palpate the right upper quadrant looking for evidence of hepatomegaly. While palpating deeply in the right upper quadrant I ask the patient to inspire deeply. I look for evidence of hepatomegaly or tenderness of the liver. I percuss and palpate in the same way in the left upper quadrant looking for evidence of splenomegaly or a ruptured spleen (in blunt trauma). I palpate the two lower quadrants as well looking for masses, fullness or tenderness.

I feel the abdominal wall looking for hernias especially if the patient has had previous abdominal surgery. There may be hernias in the previous wound repair. I check the umbilicus looking for an umbilical hernia. I auscultate the abdomen listening for bowel sounds and a possible bruit from an abdominal aortic aneurysm.

I percuss the lower abdomen between the pubis and the umbilicus looking for dullness which may indicate a distended bladder. Urinary retention is common in males with enlarged prostates and common in post operative and post traumatic settings.

*Case Study:*
*A 63 year old woman was seen in the emergency room complaining of lower abdominal pain of recent onset. The only abnormality on abdominal exam was dullness to percussion from the pubis to the umbilicus. She was unable to urinate. We were able to catheterize her to relieve a distended bladder. Further work up including an MRI disclosed a perineal tumor pressing on the urethra.*

*The only physical examination abnormality was the dullness to percussion between the pubis and the umbilicus. I saw this patient before bladder scans were available.*

I palpate the inguinal canals feeling for hernias. I ask the patient to cough feeling for a cough impulse which indicates a hernia. In male patients I push my little finger up the scrotum and into each inguinal canal. I ask the patient to cough feeling for a cough impulse which indicates a hernia.

*Case Study:*
*A patient who was on high dose steroids for an inflammatory condition came to the emergency room at the Peter Bent Brigham Hospital complaining of mild abdominal pain. The patient did not seem to be in distress. The entire abdomen felt rigid like a board with muscle spasm of the abdominal muscles. This was before MRIs and rapid CT scans. The senior surgical resident performed a paracentesis of the abdominal cavity and obtained creamy pus in the syringe. This was a case of advanced peritonitis. The normal symptoms of peritonitis were obscured by the high dose steroids. The normal symptoms and physical findings were altered by the high dose steroids.*

# CHAPTER SIXTEEN

# Examination of the Neck and Cervical Spine

First, of course, comes observation. Does the patient hold her head in a normal position? In torticollis the head is held in a slightly flexed and rotated position and the neck does not move through a full range of motion. Infants may present with a muscular torticollis. Adults also may present with similar findings.

In a setting with a history of trauma to the neck or head, the neck should be immobilized until x-rays confirm structural stability of the cervical spine. I repeat, the neck should not be moved until structural stability of the neck is confirmed by imaging studies.

Assuming the patient does not have torticollis and there is no history of trauma, I palpate the posterior muscles of the neck feeling for muscle spasm. I palpate the spinous processes looking for area of tenderness. Tenderness of the C7 spinous process may indicate clay shoveler's fracture of the C7 spinous process. I saw two cases in my career. I ask the patient to forward flex fully, extend fully, rotate right and left fully and lateral bend fully to both sides to evaluate the range of motion.

A full examination of the neck includes examining the nerves and muscles of the arms and possibly legs. This has been covered elsewhere.

To examine the thyroid, the examiner should stand behind the seated patient. Gently palpate with your fingers on both sides of the antero-lateral neck just below the thyroid cartilage. Ask the patient to swallow. An enlarged thyroid will bulge upwards more than normal.

Palpating under the jaw checks for enlarged salivary glands. Palpating along the antero-lateral neck and along the supra clavicular space examines for enlarged lymph nodes. Palpating the axillae also looks for enlarged lymph nodes.

# CHAPTER SEVENTEEN:

# Examination of the Thoracic Spine and Lumbar Spine; Gait Analysis

I always examine the thoracic and lumbar spine together. I never examine one without the other.

The physical examination should include observation of the skin as discussed previously. Observation, first. Observation, always.

*Case Study:*

*A patient was referred to an orthopedic surgeon by an internist for evaluation and treatment of low back pain. The pain had been present for about a week and was getting worse. The pain did not radiate to the legs or elsewhere. There was no numbness or tingling. As part of his low back examination protocol, one of my partners looked at the skin of the low back and sacral area. There was an obvious infected pilonidal cyst with redness, swelling and tenderness. My partner referred the patient to a general surgeon for treatment. Failure to examine the skin of the low back by the referring internist resulted in a failure to make the correct diagnosis. The low back examination protocol of the referring internist did not include examination of the skin of the low back. This is a true story.*

*Case Study:*
*A patient who had been in the intensive care unit for several weeks complained of low back pain. Orthopedic consultation was requested. Rolling the patient on her side to examine the skin of the low back as a start to the physical examination of the low back disclosed a pressure sore which had not been noticed by the physicians and nurses caring for her.*

*The physical examination and care of any bedridden patient, acute or chronic, should include daily skin checks for impending or present pressure sores. It requires time, effort and often teamwork to roll a patient to the side for a pressure sore check. Failure to perform this examination daily and at any physical examination will lead to missing impending or present pressure sores. This is a true story. I recognize that I am being preachy once again.*

Continuing the thoracic and lumbar spine examination. I perform gentle percussion of the thoracic and lumbar spine with the ulnar side of my closed fist. I am looking for any level of tenderness which might indicate a compression fracture, discitis or infection of a disc space or vertebral body. My percussion extends to the costo-vertebral angles looking for possible upper urinary tract issues which might present with a complaint of back pain.

Stance and posture are part of any physical examination of the low back and lower extremity.

There is a wide range of "normal" when examining posture. Gross observation will disclose a patient with torticollis who presents with the neck rotated and angulated. Further exam will demonstrate muscle spasm and limitation of motion of the neck with this diagnosis. An unusually short neck may suggest the possibility of Turner's Syndrome. Kyphosis of the thoracic spine is seen in patients with osteoporosis, in patients who have had thoracic vertebra fractures in the past and is sometimes congenital.

As you stand behind the patient place your hands on both shoulders. Are the shoulders level and of equal height? Uneven height of shoulders is seen in scoliosis and in patients with leg length discrepancies. Some patients have uneven height of shoulders with no other significant problem.

Place your hands on the patient's iliac crests on both sides. Are the iliac crests of equal height or are they uneven? Uneven heights of iliac crests may indicate leg length discrepancy or pelvic asymmetry.

Have the patient bend forward at the waist and look for a rib hump. Look along the spine from the inferior side toward the head. If the ribs are higher on one side, this is called a rib hump. If seen, there is a high probability the patient has scoliosis. This should be part of every physical examination of teenagers, especially girls. The earlier scoliosis is picked up the better the treatment outcome.

There are patients who have a degree of congenital thoracic kyphosis. I occasionally saw teenagers in my office who sat in a "slouched" thoracic kyphotic position. Their parents brought them in for treatment of their "bad" posture. When asked to "sit up straight" these patients are able to do so, but they are using significant contraction of the paraspinal muscles in order to do this. They are unable to maintain this straightened posture due to the continued muscular effort it requires. X-rays show a simple kyphotic curvature without other abnormality. No treatment is indicated. Counseling and acceptance are the treatment.

The lower back may have exaggerated lordosis. There is a wide range of "normal". Excessive lordosis may be seen in severe spondylolisthesis.

Observation of the upper thoracic area from the back may disclose asymmetry of the scapulae. This may indicate scoliosis. Some patients have scapular asymmetry without other significant issues.

Have the patient flex, extend the spine and perform lateral bending to both sides. Rigidity or marked limitation of motion of the spine may be seen in infection of a disc space, infection of a vertebral body, ankylosing spondylitis, diffuse idiopathic skeletal hyperostosis (DISH), lumbar strain and herniated discs among many other causes. For a problem isolated to the lumbar spine, the thoracic spine may move well while the lumber spine has limited movement. On lateral bending this will be seen with a sense of a high take off on lateral bending. This means the lateral bending occurs higher level than normal since the lumbar spine is not bending much.

Any male teenager with back pain should have his chest excursion measured. Take a measuring tape and place it around the chest at nipple level. Have the patient breathe out as much as possible and then inhale as much as possible. Measure the change in circumference of the chest. The normal change in chest circumference is often between two and four inches. Any lung disease may decrease this. A chest excursion of less than one inch, particularly in a teenaged male demands a work up for ankylosing spondylitis.

Leg Length Measurements

If the iliac crests are level there is usually no need to measure leg lengths. If the iliac crests are of uneven height then measuring leg lengths is appropriate. Palpate the anterior superior iliac spine (ASIS) on each side sequentially. Place one end of a tape measure over the ASIS. Then stretch out the tape measure and palpate the tape over the medial malleolus (MM) of the ipsilateral ankle. Do this for both sides. Next, place the end of the tape measure over the umbilicus (UMB). Then stretch out the tape and palpate over the medial malleolus of each side sequentially. A difference in the first measurement (ASIS to MM) in comparing sides suggests an actual leg length discrepancy.

You can follow up and measure the distance from the ASIS to the ipsilateral medial knee joint line (MKJL). Then measure the distance from the MKJL to the MM. This will help to determine if the difference in leg length is more from the thigh, the lower leg or both. I recall one patient with equal overall leg lengths whose femur was longer and tibial shorter than the opposite side. The result was equal leg lengths but uneven knee heights.

If the measurement from the UMB to the MM shows asymmetry while the ASIS TO MM are equal, this suggests pelvic asymmetry or angulation. A hip adduction contracture may give similar findings.

Gait

The analysis of gait is complex and can fill an entire book. In this section I present only an introduction to gait analysis. How does your patient walk? How does your patient run? The analysis of a patient's gait focuses on separately studying the stance phase of each leg and the swing phase of each leg. In a normal walking gait there is a rhythmic repetitive symmetric alternation from one leg to the other. For the ambulatory patient, I will ask the patient to walk back and forth up and down the hall. This allows enough distance to study the patient's gait.

If the patient spends less time in stance phase for one foot, this is like the "nail in the foot" gait. This is an antalgic or painful gait usually indicating a problem in the foot, ankle, lower leg or knee. This is called a shortened stance phase.

When one stands on one leg the short muscles surrounding the hip contract to hold the hip joint steady. This muscle contracture about the hip increases the pressure across the hip joint to greater than that of the body weight alone. Attempts to measure the increase in pressure across the hip joint have led to estimates of two and a half to five times body weight.

If the hip joint is painful the patient will automatically decrease pressure across the hip joint. This is accomplished by leaning the upper part of the body over the affected hip joint. If the center of gravity of the upper body is placed over the hip joint, the small muscles surrounding the hip joint do not need to contract as much to balance the body during stance phase. The instinctive limp of leaning over the affected hip decreases pressure across the hip joint in stance phase. In an antalgic hip pain gait the patient will shift his upper body over the affected hip in each stance phase of gait. This may be difficult to distinguish from a short leg gait. Measurement of leg lengths may help clarify the reason for this abnormal gait.

Why spend so much time discussing analysis of gait? Only orthopedic surgeons need to know that? Right? I say, "No!" I repeat, "No!" Why, you ask? You, the examining medical provider, should examine the gait of any teenager complaining of hip, thigh or knee pain. This is particularly important if the teenager is tall or overweight. If this teenage patient has an antalgic hip gait, check for pain on hip rotation when the patient is supine on an examining table. If any of these examination tests are abnormal, immediately make the patient non-weight bearing until x-rays are obtained to evaluate the possibility of a slipped capital femoral epiphysis (SCFE). If this is ignored, i.e. missed, the proximal capital epiphysis, may quickly slip far enough that there is long term harm to the patient.

In the course of my career as an orthopedic surgeon and hand surgeon, I saw two teenage patients who were previously evaluated by their pediatrician for hip pain. Both patients were not sufficiently evaluated initially. Neither was placed non-weight bearing and immediately sent for x-rays. Both patients had symptoms prior to a major slip. Both saw their pediatricians. Both had a chance at an early pick up. Both were missed. Both suffered long term major harm. Don't let this happen to any patient of yours. Yes, I am being preachy again. Yes, I feel strongly about this. So, should you! Don't ever miss an early slipping capital femoral epiphysis in your career!

There is a type of hip fracture in adults which occurs at the femoral neck. The bone of the femoral neck is compressed and shifts slightly into a mild valgus displacement. This fracture is temporarily stable. A patient may walk on this fracture for a few days to even a week or two before it finally falls apart. If this fracture is diagnosed acutely, it can be stabilized with a "small" operation with a small incision and stabilizing pins. If diagnosis is delayed and the fracture falls apart, then a bigger operation is needed. Also, the patient may injure himself when he falls again when the fracture comes apart.

*Case Study:*

*Years ago, I saw a patient in my office with hip pain following a fall. Examination exhibited hip pain on log rolling of the involved leg. X-rays showed a valgus impacted fracture of the femoral neck. I advised immediate hospitalization and surgery to stabilize the fracture while he healed. My patient refused surgery and walked out of my office. I saw him again a week and a half later after the fracture displaced and he fell. The corrective surgery required was the bigger operation.*

Any patient who walks with an antalgic gait following a fall and who has pain on log rolling of the hip should be evaluated with x-rays. He should be advised not to walk on the leg until the x-rays are obtained. This will prevent missing this fracture. A patient with a temporarily stable valgus impacted fracture of the hip may walk into the examining room of pretty much any medical provider. Examining a patient's gait looking for a hip antalgic gait, should be part of the physical examination toolkit of every medical provider.

A broad based gait may indicate Parkinson's disease, severe peripheral neuropathy and a multitude of other neurologic problems. A high stepping gait may indicate a peroneal palsy on the side of the high step. Classically, we were taught that a bilateral high stepping gait may indicate late syphilis. I never saw a case.

Patients walking with a bent forward posture, rigidity in movement and short steps may have Parkinson's disease or similar movement disorders. Ask these patients if they have difficulty letting go of something they are holding. If the answer is yes, consider the diagnosis of Parkinson's disease.

A wide based gait in which the feet are kept farther apart than normal is a patient's automatic reaction to difficulty with balance and movement. This is often seen with cerebellar dysfunction. Patients with severe peripheral neuropathy with or without diabetes mellitus may have dysfunctional gaits and are at high risk of injuries from falling. If examination discloses severe loss of sensation of the feet and lower legs, preventive treatment such as recommending the use of a walker to minimize the risk of falls is indicated.

Straight Leg Raising

With the patient lying on the examining table supine I gently log roll the leg as a start to my exam expecting this to be pain free. If this maneuver is not pain free I focus on examining the hip and thigh.

With one hand on the foot and the other on the knee I bend the knee ninety degrees and rotate the hip through internal and external rotation. I expect this to be pain free. If not, I focus on a detailed evaluation of the hip joint.

I perform the two maneuvers above for two reasons. One, to get the patient used to my moving his leg around. Two, to eliminate false positive straight leg raising tests which might be caused by hip or femoral pathology.

The straight leg raising test is classically performed by holding the heel of a patient's leg while the patient is supine and lifting the leg while the knee is straight. While doing this the examiner looks for evidence of pain as she elevates the leg until the hip is flexed sixty degrees. If there is pain the examiner notes at what angle of hip flexion the pain occurs.

If the straight leg raising test is positive, that is painful, then flex the hip sixty degrees and knee ninety degrees and gradually straighten the knee looking for pain before the knee is fully extended.

The two tests mentioned above are, if positive, suggestive for lower lumbar nerve root irritation possibly caused by a herniated lumbar disc at L 4-5 or L5-S1. These tests are suggestive only. As in most physical examination tests they are suggestive only and not definitive. I have deliberately described these two tests without giving them specific names. I find that if you ask five orthopedic surgeons how to perform the Laseque test, you will likely get at least three different answers. Using the names of many diagnostic tests in medicine results in ambiguity since the reader of the chart doesn't really know precisely what maneuver was performed.

There is confusion among medical providers regarding what to call these tests as well as many other clinical physical examination tests. For example, I was taught that the second test, I described, was called the Laseque sign. Yet, when I look on line I see others call the straight leg raising test the Laseque test or sign. This confusion regarding what different tests are named is general throughout the medical community. Confusion regarding naming tests is common in the medical community. I recall reading Adson's original article years ago and noting that he actually described three tests. If someone documents that she performed the "Adson test", you have no idea exactly what maneuver she performed.

In documenting tests in a medical chart, it is more accurate to describe the maneuver you performed rather than using a name to prevent confusion.

In examining patients with pain radiating to hip, perineum or testicle, the femoral stretch test looks for evidence of higher lumbar root irritation in the same way that the straight leg raising test looks for evidence of lower lumbar root irritation. For the femoral stretch test, the patient lies prone on the examining table. Bend the knee ninety degrees while holding the ankle with one hand. Place the other hand under the distal thigh and lift the distal thigh up extending the hip joint. If the patient experiences pain this is a positive test and suggestive of higher lumbar nerve root irritation but not diagnostic.

# CHAPTER EIGHTEEN:

# Examination of the Shoulder

I now move on to the musculoskeletal examination, joint by joint. Again, observation first. Always observation. Is there asymmetry? Are there skin changes (you need to remove the patient's shirt), masses, atrophy or deformity. Asymmetry may be due to the swelling of a mass or inflammation, unilateral atrophy or deformity from an acute or malunited fracture. Redness of the skin may indicate infection or calcific tendinitis. A linear vesicular lesion may indicate shingles. And so on.

In some patients there may be a sense that the humeral head is resting more distal than it should. There may be a sense of an indentation of the skin above the humeral head. This may be seen in axillary nerve palsy, brachial plexus injuries and Parsonage-Turner syndrome. Basically, this inferior subluxation is a sign of weakness of the deltoid muscle. In patients with acute fractures of the shoulder, the deltoid may temporarily relax and allow the humeral head to rest in an inferior position. This is called pseudo subluxation. I don't really like the terminology since the subluxation is real. The subluxation is temporary hence the use of the word "pseudo" I guess.

*Case Study:*

*A patient came to the orthopedic clinic complaining of right shoulder pain. This was during summer so that the skin of the right arm and shoulder were immediately obvious to observation. The right arm was red from the top of the shoulder down to the elbow. Number one in the instant observation differential diagnosis was cellulitis, given the wide extent of redness. Palpation of the red area disclosed no tenderness and no induration. Further examination showed point tenderness at the point of the shoulder and was otherwise normal in detail repeated by several orthopedic residents and an attending. X-rays showed calcific tendinitis of the right shoulder. This was an unusual presentation of calcific tendinitis of the shoulder.*

Palpation of the Shoulder

Palpation of the superficial anatomy of the shoulder includes specifically and sequentially palpating the superficial anatomic structures in a proto-col driven order. My protocol driven palpation of the shoulder includes the sterno-clavicular joint, the clavicle, the acromio-clavicular joint, the biceps tendon at the bicipital groove and the point of the shoulder. Depending on the patient's complaints my examination may extend to palpation of the scapula, for example, if there is a question of a fracture of the scapula. Tenderness in at any point requires further evaluation. Obviously, any masses noted need to be palpated.

Range of Motion of the Shoulder

For range of motion I asked the patient to raise her arms over her head moving them forward. Then I ask her to moving them out to the side over her head. Then I test extension. Then I test internal and external rotation with the arms at the side and then with the arms at 90 degrees of abduction. If the range of motion is normal, I move on. If the range of motion is not normal then more detailed testing looks at passive range of motion, sometimes with the patient supine.

Whenever there is limited active range of motion, I look to see if there is a difference between active and passive range of motion. Testing range of motion of the shoulder early and often is important. I have lost count of the number of patients for whom I have diagnosed a frozen shoulder which were missed by general medical providers, orthopedic surgeons, hand surgeons and others. Any patient who has been ill, been in the hospital, been in the ICU, had a heart attack or suffered an arm or hand injury definitely should have the range of motion of their shoulders tested early and often. Any older patient should have the range of motion of their shoulders tested. Frozen shoulders are another diagnosis I have seen missed more times than I can count. Be proactive and look for frozen shoulders. Encourage shoulder motion in patient who are hospitalized or ill to prevent frozen shoulders.

Muscle Testing

Muscle testing at the start can be performed with the patient standing or sitting. I test the deltoid by having the patient put her arms at 90 degrees of abduction and push up against gravity. Then biceps by having the patient flex the elbow to 90 degrees with the arms at her side and push up against resistance. Triceps is tested by having the patient push out against the resisting hand. While doing this I palpate the scapula with my other hand. I am feeling for winging of the scapula. With the arms at her side, I test the strength of internal and external rotation against resistance. Shoulder active internal and external rotation may be tested with the patient sitting, arms at the sides, elbows bent 90 degrees and having the patient push against resistance for internal and external rotation. Testing for rotation is more likely to show abnormalities in patients with strokes, Parsonage Turner syndrome, muscle dystrophies, rotator cuff tears and shingles of the shoulder.

If I find any weakness, I proceed to more detailed testing using the zero to five scale and looking for information which may lead me toward a diagnosis or diagnoses.

Provocative tests for the shoulder exam

Impingement test

With the patient's arm abducted 90 degrees, I passively internally and externally rotate the upper arm while palpating the acromial area with my other hand. I am feeling for a sense of crepitus under the acromion and also looking to see if this maneuver causes the patient any pain. I am looking for evidence of subacromial impingement syndrome. This test may be painful in patients with degenerative arthritis of the acromio-clavicular joint, in patients with rotator cuff tears and in patients with degenerative arthritis of the shoulder.

Test for snapping scapula syndrome

Standing behind the patient I put one hand gently over the superior medial angle of the scapula. Then, I ask the patient to circumduct the shoulder in a shrugging manner actively. I then perform circumduction passively. I am looking for a distinct snapping, rubbing or crepitus sensation under my hand at the superior medial border of the scapula. If I feel distinct snapping, rubbing or crepitus at the superior medial angle of the scapula, then this suggests possible snapping scapula syndrome.

Shoulder anterior instability test

With the upper arm abducted 90 degrees, I gently rotate the shoulder into maximum external rotation. I then gently attempt to push the shoulder into further external rotation. Some patient will express pain or a marked uncomfortable sensation. When asked some will report that it feels like their shoulder is coming out of joint. Some patients with anterior instability of the shoulder will find this maneuver quite disturbing.

Examination for possible dislocations of the shoulder

An anterior dislocation of the shoulder is fairly obvious. The humerus is abducted and externally rotated. The external rotation come from the fact that as the humeral head moves anteriorly there is a stretch placed on the external rotating muscles. This causes marked limitation of internal rotation. Even if you don't make the diagnosis of an anterior dislocation of the shoulder, you shouldn't miss the fact that there is something wrong with the shoulder which requires at the minimum x-ray imaging. The inability to elevate the arms over his head which I have discussed before will alert you that there is a shoulder problem. You can often palpate the humeral head anterior to the shoulder joint.

In posterior dislocations of the shoulder, the arm may be at the side with limitation of motion. When the humeral head moves posteriorly, there is stretch placed on the internal rotators of the shoulder. The signature finding of a posterior dislocation of the shoulder is marked limitation of external rotation. Again, the patient is unable to elevate the arm overhead. The limited elevation of the shoulder should at the minimum establish the fact that there is a shoulder problem.

In routine x-rays of normal shoulders there is often slight overlap of the humeral head and the glenoid. This is due to the fact that the shoulder (gleno-humeral) joint is angled and not facing straight forward. To obtain a "true AP" x-ray of the gleno-humeral joint radiology technicians angle the patient between 30 and 45 degrees. In a posterior dislocation of the shoulder joint a routine antero-posterior x-ray of the shoulder may only show a small degree of overlap of the humeral head and the glenoid. A posterior dislocation of the shoulder may be missed by radiologists unless either an axillary or a Y view is obtained.

The short, short is that you cannot trust routine shoulder x-rays to rule out a posterior dislocation of the shoulder. I repeat: You cannot trust routine shoulder x-rays to rule out a posterior dislocation of the shoulder. This diagnosis is commonly missed. The assumption is that the patient has a frozen shoulder. For every frozen shoulder you see, check for limited external rotation. For every shoulder you see with limited motion obtain axillary x-rays and Y view x-rays.

I repeat: The key in your examination of a shoulder with marked limitation of motion and x-rays read as normal, is to look for evidence on exam of marked limitation of external rotation. This may be the only clue to a missed posterior dislocation of the shoulder. If there is question obtain an axillary x-ray view and a Y x-ray view. Posterior dislocation of the shoulder is remarkably easy to miss.

# CHAPTER NINETEEN:

# Examination of the Elbow

---

## Observation

I check the skin for redness, swelling and skin breaks. I look for posterior swelling which may indicate an olecranon bursitis which is common. If found ask the patient if he spends time leaning on his elbow. If so, part of treatment needs to include advise to stop leaning on his elbow. I look at the angle of the elbow from the anterior direction. Childhood fractures may lead to improper growth of the distal humerus and angulation at the elbow. Excess cubitus valgus is associated with traction and ulnar nerve compression neuropathy at the elbow. If you see a patient with excess elbow valgus, evaluate the ulnar nerve with extra care.

Examine the gross shape of the upper arm. Patients with a rupture of the proximal head of the biceps will exhibit a distal shifting of the biceps muscle contour. This is common and not usually a functional or painful problem. Patients with a rupture of the distal biceps tendon will exhibit proximal migration of the belly of the biceps muscle belly. These changes may be difficult to recognize in obese patients.

On a few occasions in my career I found drainage of fluid through the skin from the posterior aspect of the elbow. The drainage was not coming from the olecranon bursa, which would be a natural first assumption, but from the elbow joint itself. These few patients had severe rheumatoid arthritis. The drainage was coming from a synovial bursal fistula draining into the olecranon bursa from the elbow joint and then through a bursal cutaneous fistula through the skin.

I also look for generalized swelling of the elbow joint which might indicate an inflammatory synovitis, a crystal induced synovitis or an infectious synovitis. And as always, I look for masses.

Palpation

Once again, I move from proximal to distal and medial to lateral as part of my "easy" to remember superficial anatomy palpation protocol. If indicated I palpate the upper arm. If there is a complaint of pain in the upper arm, there may be soft tissue masses, bone tumors, nerve tumors, etc. Otherwise, as I take the elbow in my hands I feel for warmth, joint effusion and a separate olecranon bursal effusion. Olecranon bursal effusions are common. Note: any location of tenderness may indicate an underlying fracture.

In sequence, I palpate the medial epicondyle looking for tenderness which might indicate medial epicondylitis. I palpate the ulnar nerve at the cubital tunnel looking for tenderness which might indicate cubital tunnel syndrome. While palpating the medial epicondyle gently, I flex and extend the elbow looking for anterior subluxation of the ulnar nerve at the elbow. I continue with palpation of the lateral epicondyle looking for tenderness which might indicate lateral epicondylitis also called tennis elbow. I palpate the radial head. Tenderness may indicate a fracture of the radial head. I then palpate the radial nerve at the radial tunnel. Radial tunnel syndrome is rare and difficult to diagnose with confidence. Many patients have a mild degree of tenderness over the radial tunnel which is not clinically significant. If I find tenderness at the radial tunnel, I compare with palpation on the other side. Often the mild tenderness at the radial tunnel is equal bilaterally. Asymmetry in tenderness at the radial tunnel or greater tenderness than expected at the radial tunnel increases the possibility of radial tunnel syndrome in a patient with complaints of non-specific pain in the arm.

Range of Motion

I ask the patient to bend and straighten the elbow fully. I do the same for pronation and supination. If there is limited active motion, I check to see if the active and passive motions are the same.

Provocative Tests

If there is question of stability of the ligaments of the elbow joint, hold the back of the elbow gently with one hand with the elbow extended, then exert mild to moderate pressure trying to move the forearm in a radial and ulnar direction looking for varus or valgus motion which the patient should not exhibit.

Performing the Tinel's sign at the cubital tunnel, that is tapping the ulnar nerve at the cubital tunnel looks for evidence of irritation of the ulnar nerve and possible cubital tunnel syndrome.

# CHAPTER TWENTY

# The Physical Examination of the Wrist and Hand

The wrist and hand are so close to each other anatomically and intermingled and intertwined with each other that I present them together. I never examine the wrist without examining the hand and I never examine the hand without examining the wrist.

Observation

Is the skin normal color? Any area of redness may indicate inflammation from infection, inflammatory arthritis or crystal induced inflammation in a joint or in the soft tissue. Are there small dots in an area of redness which might indicate an insect or spider bite. In my practice these were most common on the dorsum of the hand. Black areas on the fingertips may be areas of necrosis from decreased blood supply. Are any of the fingers unusually white indicative of Raynaud's phenomenon or Raynaud's disease.

Do the fingers look normal? Clawing of the ring and little finger may indicate an ulnar nerve palsy. Zigzag deformities of multiple fingers may indicate severe systemic lupus erythematosus or rheumatoid arthritis. A mass on the dorsum of the wrist is likely a ganglion, but not always. A small mass on the dorsum of the distal interphalangeal joint may indicate a mucous cyst which is another name for a ganglion on the dorsum of that joint. A slightly irregular mass on a finger may be a giant cell tumor of tendon sheath. These continue to grow in size and have a propensity to recur after surgical excision. The larger the mass the greater the likelihood for recurrence. Any mass on a finger should be evaluated by a hand surgeon.

Is the resting position of the fingers normal? If a flexor tendon is cut the involved finger will likely rest in a straighter position than normal. If an extensor tendon is cut the finger or part of the finger will likely droop palmarward greater than normal. The area and nature of droop will depend on the level of the cut tendon. An extensor tendon cut at the wrist or dorsal hand will cause the finger to droop at the metacarpal phalangeal joint. If cut dorsal to the proximal phalanx the finger will droop at the proximal interphalangeal joint. If cut or ruptured at the level of the middle phalanx or distal interphalangeal joint only the distal joint will droop, called a mallet finger. If the thumb extensor tendon has been cut or if it ruptures spontaneously the thumb will hang down more when the hand is held in the air palm down.

This quick evaluation of the resting position of the fingers and thumb are an important part of the evaluation of any patient who has suffered a skin break of the hand or wrist. If you are evaluating a patient who has previously been seen in an emergency room or walk in clinic you need to double check that a lacerated tendon and/or lacerated nerve was not missed.

A quick evaluation for rupture or laceration of the extensor tendon of the thumb follows: ask the patient to place her hand palm down on a table. While keeping the palm touching the table, ask the patient to lift here thumb up off of the table. If the thumb extensor tendon is lacerated or ruptured she will be unable to elevate the thumb up off of the table.

Is there atrophy of the intrinsic muscles of the hand? This is exhibited by deeper concavities between the metacarpal bones. This finding is more common as the age of the patient examined increases. Does the contour of the base of the thumb at the carpo-metacarpal joint look normal? Does the base of the first metacarpal look like it is subluxing out of joint radially? Is the first metacarpal lying next to the second metacarpal in an adducted position?

Palpation of finger tips for hydrosis. If there is normal peripheral nerve function, the finger tips will have "mild" sweating and friction will be sensed when you rub your finger tip across the patient's fingertip. If nerve function to the fingertip is interrupted, there is no innervation of the sweat glands in the finger tips. The skin of the finger tips will be smooth and dry. There will be decreased resistance when you rub you your finger across the patient's injured fingertip. With normal innervation of the fingertip, the skin of the fingertip is more moist and is not smooth and dry.

Any evaluation of the wrist should include a quick examination of the shoulder and elbow. As in all upper extremity examinations, if my examination is oriented toward the wrist, I ask the patient to raise their arms over their head for a quick evaluation of the range of motion of the shoulder. This also allows me a quick evaluation of how the patient moves their upper extremities.

I take the forearm and wrist in my hands and gently palpate the mid-radius noticing how the patient responds to gentle palpation in an area I do not expect to be tender. Obviously, if I think there may be an injury or fracture of the forearm, I start differently. I position the wrist with the thumb up. My protocol driven palpation and provocative test physical examination of the wrist and hand tends to run from proximal to distal and radial to ulnar. Having palpated the mid-radius without a response, I may tap the mid radius for a Tinel's sign which I expect to be negative. I am performing a quick initial evaluation of the patient's reactivity and/or symptom magnification. I am establishing a baseline for how my patient reacts to palpation in an area I do not expect to be tender.

I next palpate the first dorsal extensor compartment (1DEC). Tenderness may indicate DeQuervain's stenosing tenosynovitis (DEQ). This used to be common in secretaries who did a lot of filing in their work. Now, I find it most common in newborn mothers either from the newer breast feeding positions in which the mother holds the baby with the wrist fully volar flexed or from the method of holding the heavy baby carriers currently in use. I also palpate the 1DEC feeling for small one to three millimeter firm masses which are usually small ganglions of tendon sheath of the 1DEC. I have the patient put his thumb into the palm and place the fingers around the thumb. Holding the fingers around the thumb, I gently passively ulnar deviate the wrist. This is called the Finkelstein test. Pain at the first dorsal extensor compartment with this maneuver suggests DeQuervains tendinitis.

The differential diagnosis for a positive Finkelstein test includes Dequervain's stenosing tenosynovitis, fracture of the distal radius, fracture or non-union of a fracture of the scaphoid, radio-carpal wrist joint degenerative arthritis, scaphoid-trapezium-trapezoid degenerative arthritis and thumb carpo-meta-carpal degenerative arthritis. These diagnoses are all possible causes of radial wrist pain and tenderness. I gently try to volar flex the wrist and see if the thumb easily, passively touches the volar forearm. This is a quick and easy test to see if the patient has generally loose ligaments or tight ligaments.

Next, I palpate of the anatomic snuff box looking for tenderness. I find it useful to ulnar deviate the wrist while doing this. I am able to present the scaphoid so that I am able to palpate the scaphoid specifically. If I find snuff box tenderness, I palpate the opposite side for comparison. Occasional patients exhibit mild tenderness which is equal bilaterally and which is not pathologic. Tenderness of the snuff box suggests possible fracture or non-union of a fracture of the scaphoid. Non displaced fractures of the scaphoid may be missed on routine x-rays of the wrist. Other diagnoses presenting with tenderness of the snuff box to palpation include avascular necrosis of the scaphoid with micro cortical fracture, degenerative arthritis of the radio-carpal wrist which may be isolated to the radio scaphoid joint and the other diagnoses listed above for a positive Finkelstein test.

Next, I palpate the first carpo-metacarpal joint, also called the basal thumb joint, also called the trapezium-first metacarpal joint. I look for tenderness and deformity, specifically radial subluxation of the base of the first meta-carpal, both of which are characteristic of basal thumb arthritis also called thumb carpo-metacarpal arthritis (CMCJ DJD). If I find evidence for CMCJ DJD I evaluate the motion of the thumb looking for evidence of adduction contracture of the thumb seen in later stages of CMC DJD.

Can the patient actively or passively elevate the thumb out of the palm called opposition? Can the patient grasp a normal size glass with normal opening of the thumb and fingers? If there is an adduction contracture of the thumb, I check for radial laxity of the metacarpal phalangeal joint (MPJ). At late stages of CMCJ DJD the ulnar collateral ligament of the metacarpal phalangeal joint of the thumb ruptures due to repetitive strain and the MPJ develops radial instability weakening grip.

Even if the exam of the CMCJ is normal, my wrist and hand examination moves on to evaluation of the MPJ of the thumb. The evaluation of every injury of the thumb should include testing of the stability of the MPJ of the thumb. With the joint in full extension gently move the proximal phalanx in a radial and ulnar direction looking for laxity. Then flex the MPJ 30 degrees and again test for radial and ulnar laxity.

In complete ruptures of the ulnar collateral ligament (UCL) the proximal phalanx will move 60 degrees or more with gentle radial stress when the joint is in 30 degrees of flexion. If you test for this routinely you will find occasional patients with chronic rupture of the UCL who know that their thumb is weak but are not complaining about it. Complete rupture of the UCL of the MPJ of the thumb is called Gamekeeper's thumb. Instability in the ulnar direction implies rupture of the radial collateral ligament of the MPJ of the thumb.

Complete rupture of the collateral ligaments of the thumb is one of the more commonly missed diagnoses which I saw in my office. The diagnosis was missed in emergency rooms (ER), and offices of family medicine physicians and internists. Missing this diagnosis results in the patient requiring a different reconstructive operation if recognition is delayed.

In the 37 ½ years of my practice I operated on numerous patients with instability of this joint following an "acute" injury. I estimate that ten percent of these patients at surgery had no evidence of an acute injury. Instead they had a recent minor sprain of the thumb on top of an old, unrecognized Gamekeeper's thumb. For my preoperative counseling for all of these patients I told them that there was a ten percent chance I would need to do the operation for chronic Gamekeeper's thumb rather than the operation for acute Gamekeeper's thumb.

I repeat, this diagnosis is often missed. For any injury involving the thumb, every physical examination should include a specific evaluation of the possibility of this injury. If you find laxity of the ligaments, this may be new or old.

Continuing my exam, I rotate the hand so that it is palm up. I observe for skin color, swelling masses and the resting position of the hand and fingers. I swipe my thumb gently across the palm feeling for cords of Dupuytren's contracture. I often find Dupuytren's cords in patients who are not complaining about it. If I find evidence of Dupuytren's contracture, I shift to a family history of Dupuytren's as well as looking for a family history of Scottish, English or Irish ancestry.

I look for redness, swelling, masses. I palpate the palm a little deeper so that the patient is comfortable with my pressure which does not cause pain. I palpate the A1 pulleys of the thumb and four fingers. I also feel for a small 1-3 mm firm mass which usually indicates a ganglion of tendon sheath of the flexor tendon sheath at the A1 pulley. Tenderness over the A1 pulleys may indicate tenosynovitis or trigger fingers or thumb. I find this diagnosis is often missed because the examining medical provider does not bother to palpate the A1 pulleys. Again, the examining provider's hand examination protocol does not include palpation of the A1 pulleys.

I palpate the pisiform and the hook of the hamate. Rare patients have "painful pisiform syndrome" or a ganglio of the hamate – pisiform joint. Others have a fracture or a non-union of a fracture of the hook of the hamate. I perform an Allen's test of the radial and ulnar arteries at the wrist. This will pick up cases of obstruction of the radial artery seen occasionally after use of a radial artery line in an ICU and also cases of hypothenar hammer syndrome with blockage of the ulnar artery at Guyon's canal. I perform the Tinel's sign test at the carpal canal and Guyon's canal.

I have the patient make a fist looking for rotatory deformity of the fingers. This is especially important in evaluating trauma to the hand. A fracture of a metacarpal or proximal or middle phalanx may displace in a rotatory fashion causing the injured finger to cross over a normal finger with fist making. Rotatory displacement of fractures of the hand is another of the frequent, and I do mean frequent, missed injuries in emergency room and outpatient office settings. This needs to be specifically looked for or it will be missed. The quick exam is to ask the patient to make a fist. If the patient makes a normal fist easily then rotation of the metacarpals and phalanges is fine.

I have the patient extend her fingers fully. I gently grasp the finger with my index, middle and ring finger on the dorsum of the finger and my thumb on the volar side of the middle phalanx. I gently hold the proximal interphalangeal joint straight and ask the patient to flex the distal interphalangeal joint. If the patient flexes the finger normally, fine. If not, is there limited motion or no motion of the distal interphalangeal joint? I do this for the thumb and four fingers. If the patient is unable to flex the tip of a digit at all, this may indicate: a lacerated flexor digitorum profundus or flexor pollicis longus tendon (old or recent), avulsion of the profundus tendon, rupture of the flexor tendon, direct muscle injury, nerve injury (acute or chronic), central nervous system abnormalities such as a stroke and lack of patient cooperation.

Failure to test for lacerations of the profundus tendons following any skin break (even the most trivial seeming puncture wound) in the hand may lead to missing a lacerated profundus tendon. This is another commonly missed injury. A penetrating injury with a sharp object which causes only a tiny laceration in the finger, hand or forearm may lacerate a tendon completely or partially or cut a nerve completely or partially.

In the absence of a skin break, profundus tendons may avulse. A common avulsion is the rugger jersey injury. Make a fist with all of your fingers. While holding your fist gently, actively closed sequentially open each finger and then pull it back in. You will find that you are able to open your index, middle and little fingers almost all of the way. You will find that your ring finger opens much less and the tip remains hooked if you maintain your fist with the other fingers. If someone grabs an object, often a part of a sweatshirt or jersey and the other person pulls away. If only the ring finger ends up holding on to the jersey then the force on the tip of the hooked ring finger may avulse the profundus tendon. The tendon pulls proximally and there is often tenderness and swelling near the proximal interphalangeal joint. This is yet another commonly missed diagnosis. For any injured finger, especially an injured ring finger, testing for active flexion of the profundus tendon at the distal interphalangeal joint is important.

In patients with rheumatoid arthritis a detailed examination for ruptured tendons is important. These ruptures are almost always pain free. Patients with severe rheumatoid arthritis are so used to impaired function of their hands that they often do not realized that a tendon has ruptured. This needs to be specifically looked for. If a patient with severe rheumatoid arthritis has a ruptured tendon, more tendons will rupture unless quickly treated. The most common first tendon ruptures are the extensor digiti quinti on the dorsum of the hand and the flexor pollicis longus on the volar side of the hand.

All of the frequently missed diagnoses I discussed above lead to worse outcomes if not diagnosed early. All of the frequently missed diagnoses I discussed above were missed due to inadequate and incomplete physical examinations. All of the frequently missed diagnoses I discussed above occurred because the examining medical providers did not utilize sufficiently thorough examination protocols.

For a patient who complains of weakness of the hand, particularly pinch testing for flexion of the profundus tendons of the thumb and index finger may show weakness. This is an uncommon problem. Chronic pressure on the anterior interosseous nerve may cause weakness of only the profundus tendons of the thumb and index finger. Very rarely, there is weakness only of the thumb flexor.

I repeat: Patients with chronic rheumatoid arthritis need to be tested for tendon ruptures frequently. Tendon ruptures in patients with rheumatoid arthritis are usually painless. On immediate gross observation, do the ulnar fingers, particularly the little finger, seem to lag full extension? On the extensor side, extensor tendon ruptures usually start on the ulnar side and progress toward the radial side. Thus, the first tendon to rupture is often the extensor digiti quinti (EDQ). The little finger has two extensor tendons, the EDQ and the extensor digitorum communis to the little finger. The EDQ may rupture without symptoms and without the patient becoming aware of this rupture. Any examination of a patient with rheumatoid arthritis should include testing of the continuity of the EDQ. Ask the patient to make a fist. Then while keeping the index, middle and ring finger in the fist position, have the patient attempt to extend the little finger at the metacarpal phalangeal joint (MCPJ). If the little finger lags and does not fully extend at the MCPJ then the EDQ may be ruptured. If this is so, the other tendons are at risk and surgery is indicated to remove the dorsally protruding distal ulna, clean out the inflamed synovium and repair and support the extensor tendons as appropriate.

On the flexor side the most common tendon to rupture and the first to rupture is often the flexor pollicis longus (FPL). The patient may only complain of weakness in the thumb. Specific examination for function of the FPL is indicated. If the FPL is ruptured and ignored there will be progression to further flexor tendon ruptures and significant loss of hand function.

Many patients complain of locking of their fingers. You may see the patient with the finger flexed and he is unable to actively straighten it. It will usually straighten passively with a little pressure. Usually you will find tenderness at the A1 pulley of the involved finger. Often you will feel a bump moving proximally and distally as you passively flex and extend the involved finger. This is swelling of the flexor tendon. This is the common trigger finger.

For all patients with locking of their fingers turn the hand palm down and ask them to slowly open and close their hand. Look carefully at the extensor tendon as it travels over the metacarpal phalangeal joint. Some patients with locking of their fingers have subluxation of the extensor tendon to the ulnar side of the metacarpal phalangeal joint of that finger. Occasional patients have ulnar subluxation of multiple extensor tendons at the metacarpal phalangeal joint. I see this more frequently in patients with lax ligaments. When patients have locking fingers from subluxation of the extensor tendon, the finger will tend to lock is a straight position rather than a curled partial fist position.

The wrist joint is a complex bundle of bones. There are numerous ways for this bundle of bones to demonstrate instability. A detailed discussion of the provocative tests for wrist instability is beyond the scope of this book.

# CHAPTER TWENTY ONE

# Physical Examination
# of the Hip

The start of the physical examination of the hip and the full examination of the hip depends on the patient's presentation to you, the medical provider.

Physical Examination of the Acutely Non-Ambulatory Adult Patient

Usually you will see an acutely non-ambulatory patient following a fall. Note that some elderly patients actually seem to break their hip and then fall. You may encounter the patient in an emergency room lying on a stretcher.

First, observation. Always, observation. Is the patient unconscious? Is the patient awake and alert? Does the patient have a vacant look? The issues of evaluating the unconscious patient determining cognitive status of the conscious patient have previously been covered. The issue of determining cognitive status is important in any trauma situation and in any evaluation of an elderly patient.

For a patient complaining of hip or leg pain, pull back the sheet and look at the legs. Observation should include examining the skin for evidence of trauma and for evidence of vascular insufficiency. Does the leg lie in a normal position? Following a fall in a patient who is unable to ambulate, the painful leg may lie in a shortened, externally rotated position. This may indicate a hip fracture of the intertrochanteric area, subtrochanteric area, a fracture of the shaft of the femur and possible hip dislocation with or without fracture. Fractures of the neck of the femur do not usually present with shortening and external rotation of the lower leg.

Gentle logrolling of each leg will help determine if there is a fracture of one or both legs.

*Case Study:*
*One of my orthopedic partners was called to the emergency room to see a patient who fell in her kitchen. She was unable to walk and complained of pain in both hips. She weighed over 400 pounds. It is difficult to perform a comprehensive physical examination in someone that size. Even observation offered limited information about the hips. Range of motion of most joints will be decreased due to the size of the arms and legs. Gentle logrolling disclosed pain in both legs. X-rays disclosed fractures of both hips.*

If a patient is determined to have a hip fracture or femur fracture, the physical examination should also check neurologic function of the legs, vascularity of the legs and the patient's general medical status for determination of best treatment.

Chronic non-ambulatory patients may have severe osteoporosis of their legs due to the lack of weight bearing. Fractures, especially femur fractures, may occur from simple handling of the patient. If logrolling causes pain, the leg needs further evaluation including x-rays.

There are other causes of a patient becoming suddenly non-ambulatory of sudden onset including strokes, brain tumor, pelvic fractures, Guillian-Barre Syndrome, shingles of the hip area (I have seen one case). Further medical history and physical exam will help to distinguish the possibilities.

Physical Examination of the Ambulatory Hip Pain Patient

First, observation. Always, observation. All patients complaining of hip pain should have their thoracic and lumbar spines examined. Pathology in the lumber spine often causes pain radiating to the posterior hip and thigh. Examination of the thoracic and lumbar spine have previously been discussed. After I have examined the patient's thoracic and lumbar spine while standing, I move on to the standing part of the hip exam.

Trendelenburg Test

While standing behind the patient with your hands placed gently on the iliac crests bilaterally, have the patient sequentially stand on each leg. If the iliac crest on the lifted leg side drops down this suggests weakness of the hip abductor muscle (gluteus medius) of the hip on the side of the planted leg. This may be seen with pain in the hip from osteoarthritis, valgus impacted hip fracture, Legg Calve Perthes disease, slipped capital femoral epiphysis, congenital dislocation of the hip, degenerative arthritis of the hip, loose hip protheses and other pain causing hip pathologies.

Weakness of hip abductors used to be an issue in post polio patients. It is important to test for hip abductor strength in patients following hip surgery for hip fracture or total hip replacement. If abductor weakness is noted the patient should be referred for therapy to increase the strength of the hip abductors. If a patient fails to regain hip abductor strength following hip injury or surgery, she is at greater risk of falling.

I repeat: A positive Trendelenburg test on the examination of a teenager who is complaining of hip pain demands immediate non-weight bearing status and x-rays to evaluate for slipped capital femoral epiphysis.

Logrolling

I briefly covered logrolling above when discussing the non-ambulatory hip patient. With a patient supine, logrolling of the leg using the foot or lower leg just rotates the hip joint unless of course the foot or lower leg is painful where you are touching. A grimace of the patient's face will indicate whether this maneuver is causing pain. Of course, in a verbal patient you can ask if the maneuver causes pain. With a patient sitting, moving the foot left and right also rotates the hip joint and is another method of examining the hip joint for pain, assuming the patient is able to sit. Pain on logrolling may indicate a problem with the hip joint. Possible diagnoses were enumerated just above. A fracture of the pubic and ischial rami of the pelvis may show pain on logrolling of the ipsilateral leg.

*Case Study:*
*In orthopedic groups, the orthopedic surgeon who operates on a hip fracture may not see the patient until just before surgery. Hip fractures are often operated on at night after the elective surgical schedule is finished. The operating surgeon is the one who is on call that night. This case was told to me by the scrub nurse and the circulating nurse who were in the operating room when this happened. I believe the story is true.*

*The orthopedic surgeon came to the hospital to operate on a patient with a hip fracture who had been admitted to the hospital by one of this orthopedic surgeon's partners. The patient was elderly and suffered from severe dementia. In the operating room the orthopedic surgeon was careful prior to surgery. He pointed to the x-rays which showed the hip fracture. He announced to all member of the operating team which side was fractured based on the labelling of the x-rays. The patient was positioned with that side up in preparation for the surgery. Just prior to making the surgical incision the orthopedic surgeon again confirmed that all operating personnel agreed he was operating on the correct side based on the x-rays.*

*The orthopedic surgeon operated and opened a normal hip joint without a fracture. He recognized that he had operated on the wrong side. He closed the incision and then turned the patient over and operated on the correct side where he found the fracture.*

*The problem? The x-rays were marked incorrectly. The sides were reversed.*

*How might this orthopedic surgeon have avoided this problem? Had the orthopedic surgeon utilized log rolling to examine this patient briefly before surgery, he could have established which side was fractured by noting pain with log rolling on one side but not the other. With repeat x-rays he could have established the fact that the original x-rays were mislabeled prior to surgery. Log rolling is a useful part of the lower extremity examination.*

*Case Study:*
*A 28 year old woman came into my office complaining of pain in her right hip. She walked with a mild limp. Logrolling performed when she was distracted clearly demonstrated pain with grimacing. X-rays of the hip joint and pelvis were normal. Detailed history disclosed unprotected sex during the previous four months. My provisional diagnosis was gonococcal septic arthritis of the right hip joint. It is difficult to obtain joint fluid samples from the hip joint for culture. I treated her with antibiotics which covered gonococcal infection and she responded quickly. A positive logrolling test of her right hip allowed me to make this diagnosis quickly. While I am unable to prove this was a gonococcal infection of the hip joint, I feel this diagnosis was likely.*

*Case Study:*

*A 2 ½ year old child comes to the emergency room crying and holding his left hip partly flexed. Gentle rotation of the affected leg clearly causes increased painful. Further work up confirms the presumptive diagnosis of septic arthritis of the hip.*

Range of motion

With the patient supine, ask her to fully flex her hip. Is she able to do this? Does the opposite leg elevate some as the hip is fully flexed. If the opposite leg lifts somewhat, ask the patient to fully flex both hips so that the knees come up to the chest. Then hold one leg fully flexed with one hand and try to fully extend the other leg. If the other leg does not fully extend, this patient has a flexion contracture of the leg you are trying to extend.

With the hip flexed 90 degrees and with the hip fully extended measure amount of internal rotation and external rotation. If there is limited internal range of motion in a teenager, the patient may have a slipped capital femoral epiphysis. Rotation of the hip joint is limited in osteoarthritis and other hip pathologies.

Thigh and Knee Examination

My physical examination protocol for the thigh and knee generally moves proximal to distal and medial to lateral. Any thigh exam should include evaluation of the hip as well. Any knee exam should at least include a logrolling maneuver looking for hip pathology and evaluation of the thigh. Hip pathology may occasionally present with only the complaint of knee pain.

Observation, first. Observation, always. Observation includes the basics of redness, swelling, masses, deformity and atrophy. I look for a sense of angulation of the knee, that is, the angle between the thigh and the lower leg, i.e. varus and valgus, which is greater than normal. In a child excessive varus or valgus angulation at the knee may indicate a congenital or developmental problem. In the adult, excessive varus or valgus of the knee may indicate degenerative arthritis which has worn away bone either on the medial or lateral side. Excessive varus or valgus may be due to other developmental problems such as childhood rickets or damage to a growth plate from childhood injury.

In teenagers complaining of distal medial thigh pain, palpation of the distal, medial thigh at the distal femoral metaphysis occasionally picks up a firm, boney mass which is a protruding osteochondroma.

Decreased thigh circumference is often seen in athletes and non-athletes following an injury to the lower leg or surgery to the lower leg. If an athlete returns to competition before rehabilitating his quadriceps muscle to normal circumference she is at greater risk of suffering another injury.

I palpate the knee for warmth and effusion. I test for effusion by placing one hand over the suprapatellar pouch. With the other hand I place my thumb on one side of the knee just posterior to the edge of the patella and the fingers of that hand on the other side of the patella. Then, I alternately gently squeeze the fingers and thumb of one hand and then the other. While doing this I feel for a sense of a fluid wave with the non-squeezing hand.

I palpate looking for specific areas of tenderness. In my protocol driven palpation exam, I palpate in order: the patella, medial retinaculum, the medial collateral ligament including origin, mid-portion and insertion. With the knee bent I palpate the medial knee joint line, anterior, middle and posterior, the inferior pole of the patella, the pes anserinus bursa, the tibial tubercle, the lateral joint line, anterior, middle and posterior and the lateral collateral ligament, proximal, middle and distal. Note: The middle portion of the collateral ligaments overlaps the middle of the knee joint lines. Note also. Palpating the pes anserinus bursa is also palpating the medial proximal tibia.

I palpate the popliteal fossa with the knee slightly bent looking for tenderness and fluctuance indicative of a popliteal (Baker's) cyst. Usually the cyst has to be large to be felt.

Isolated fluctuance anterior to the patella may indicate a patellar bursitis. Fluctuance anterior to the tibial tubercle may indicate a prepatellar bursitis. These need to be distinguished from an effusion in the knee joint itself. Fluctuance on both sides of the patella indicates a joint effusion. Tenderness at the origin or insertion of the medial collateral ligament may indicate traumatic tearing of the ligament. Tenderness at the mid-medial collateral ligament is tenderness at the mid-medial knee joint line. This may indicate a mechanical derangement in the knee, degenerative arthritis or a tear of the mid portion of the medial collateral ligament.

Tenderness at the pes anserinus may indicate a pes anserinus bursitis or a tibial plateau fracture. Pes anserinus bursitis is not a common finding. However, if you don't palpate the pes anserinus as a routine part of your exam you will occasionally miss this diagnosis. Tenderness at the inferior pole of the patella is an uncommon finding. Tenderness of the inferior pole of the patella may indicate a fracture of the patella if there has been acute trauma. Otherwise tenderness of the inferior pole of the patella may indicate jumper's knee. If you don't palpate the inferior pole of the patella as part of your routine knee exam you will miss diagnosing the occasional jumper's knee.

Palpation of the anterior and posterior lateral knee joint lines may show tenderness. The possible diagnoses are similar to the diagnoses for tenderness of the medial knee joint line. Careful palpation of the anterior part of the lateral joint line may show a localized area of fluctuance. This is seen in lateral meniscal cysts. Tenderness of the origin and insertion of the lateral collateral ligament may indicate a traumatic tear of the lateral collateral ligament. Palpation of the middle of the lateral collateral ligament at the middle of the lateral knee joint line may indicate a lateral collateral ligament tear, a mechanical derangement or degenerative arthritis.

I ask the patient to move the knee through a full range of motion and note any limitation. If there is a limit to active motion, I then test gentle passive range of motion. Are active motion and passive motion the same or is passive motion greater than active motion? Active motion should never be greater than passive motion. If you were to note that active motion was greater than passive motion then there are issues of patient compliance with the exam. If active motion is less than passive motion I move on to detailed muscle testing.

Provocative Tests

With the knee straight and the patient lying on the examining table, I grasp the patella and move it gently around so that the patient is used to my manipulating the patella gently. I then push down on the patella and move it proximally and distally. I am looking for two possibilities. I am looking to see if this maneuver causes the patient pain. I am also feeling for the vibration sense in my examining fingers which indicates crepitus. This test is called the patella-femoral grind test. Pain with the maneuver in a young patient may indicate patellar femoral pain syndrome, sometimes called chondromalacia patellae. In an older patient this may indicate patellar femoral degenerative arthritis. This obviously would be painful in a patient with a fracture of the patella. If there is a fracture of the patella, simple palpation of the patella will disclose sufficient tenderness that the examining physician should not be attempting the patellar femoral grind test.

With the patient lying supine on the examining table gently press the patella in a lateral direction. Evaluate if there is lateral subluxation of the patella and how much. The patient may experience pain and "unhappiness" and she may even sit up and grasp her knee. This is the patella apprehension test. If the patient expresses pain or distinct unhappiness with your maneuver the patellar apprehension test is positive. This may indicate ligamentous instability of the restraining ligaments and may confirm a suspicion of lateral patellar instability. Pushing the patella medially and palpating the undersurface of the patella may help confirm patella femoral pain syndrome if this elicits pain. I once had a patient who had a positive patellar apprehension sign to medial displacement of the patella. This patient had previous surgery which overcorrected her lateral patellar instability.

If there is marked laxity in lateral subluxation of the patella, especially if this is not painful, then further evaluation of general ligamentous laxity is indicated looking for variants of Ehlers Danlos Syndrome.

One test for meniscal tears is the McMurray test. With the knee bent about 90 degrees, rotate the tibial back and forth gently, then hyperflex the knee, externally rotate the tibia and slowly extend the knee looking for pain or catching. If this is painful or catches it suggests a torn meniscus. This is a "classic" knee exam test. Personally, I did not find this test useful.

Ligament stability tests

With the knee straight push the tibial gently into varus and valgus. I found the best way to test this is: let's say I am examining the right knee. I sit on the right side of the patient. I take the right ankle with my right hand. I move so that the lateral aspect of the patient's right knee is resting against the left side of my waist. I place my left hand on the medial aspect of the patient's right knee with my thumb resting on the mid portion of the medial knee joint line. I find that flexing the knee a little back and forth helps me to clearly define the medial knee joint line.

Then, with my right hand I gently pull the right ankle outwards, placing a valgus stress on the patient's right knee. With my left thumb I feel to see if the right medial knee joint line opens up. With the knee straight there should be little if any opening. If there is opening of the medial knee joint line, I document the number of millimeters of opening. I feel to see if there is a distinct stop to the opening or if the knee seems to open without a distinct stop.

I then bend the knee 30 degrees and repeat the same test. I again feel for opening of the medial knee joint line. Some patients with ligamentous laxity may have a small degree of opening without indicating pathologic ligamentous instability. Opening of 5-7 mm with a distinct stop may indicate a grade II tear of the medial collateral ligament. This is a partial tear in which the ligament is stretched but not completely torn. Opening of 10 mm or more particularly without a distinct stop indicates a complete tear of the medial collateral ligament and probably other ligaments.

The examination of the lateral collateral ligament is the mirror image of the description above. In acute injuries complete tears of the collateral ligaments and other ligaments tend to be less painful during ligament stress examination than partial tears. The reason is that in a partial tear the stress pulls on the torn ligament which hurts. If the ligament tear is complete, the stress test does not actually pull on the completely torn ligament.

With the knee straight on the examining table I place my left hand on the anterior aspect of the patient's distal thigh and press gently down. With my right hand I grasp the tibial plateau and pull upward (anteriorly). I look to see if the proximal tibial translates anteriorly on the distal femur. If there is distinct anterior translation of the tibia this may indicate a torn anterior cruciate ligament. This is the Lachmann test. I found this test useful.

I then examine the patient with the knee hanging over the edge of the examining table. I place the patient's foot on my thigh to support it. I then grasp the tibial plateau with both hands and gently pull it toward me. This is the anterior drawer sign. Pushing posteriorly is the posterior drawer sign.

There are other physical examination tests for the knee. The ones I have described are sufficient for the scope of this book.

Lower extremity muscle testing was covered in the section on muscle testing.

# CHAPTER TWENTY TWO

# The Physical Examination of the Lower Leg, Ankle and Foot

I never examine the foot without examining the ankle and I never examine the ankle without examining the foot. Like the hand and wrist, the ankle and foot are close together and intermingled, intertwined.

Observation, first. Observation, always. Is the skin normal? Is the skin red? Is there deformity or angulation of the leg? Are there ulcers suggesting vascular issues? Is there localized swelling or generalized edema?

*Case Study:*
*I am walking in a park with my family. We see an elderly man sitting on the ground holding his leg by the tibial plateau. The lower half of his lower leg is hanging down at a 60 degree angle with bone sticking out of the skin. Making the diagnosis of compound fractures of the tibia and fibula is quite easy. I introduce myself and offer my assistance. He has already called for an ambulance and declines my offer of assistance.*

Evaluating the lower leg for phlebitis involves looking for swelling and palpating for tenderness. Measurement of the maximum calf circumference will document the extent of swelling. Palpating the calf for tenderness is another part of the exam. Unfortunately, the physical examination looking for possible phlebitis is near worthless. I ordered Doppler studies on any patient complaining of leg pain for which there was no other obvious cause. I had patients with entirely normal lower leg exams whose Doppler tests were positive for phlebitis. I had patients with unilateral swelling of the lower leg and calf tenderness whose Doppler tests were negative for phlebitis. If the possibility of phlebitis enters your mind, order the test. Do not, do not, do not depend on the physical exam for determining the probability of phlebitis.

Ankle and Foot

Again. Observation, first. Observation, always. Is there swelling of one or both ankles. If there is swelling of both ankles, more or less equally, is there pitting edema of the ankles? Redness, especially red streaks may indicate cellulitis or lymphangitis.

What is pitting edema? Edema by definition is swelling of the tissues caused by increased fluid in the tissues rather than from a mass. In examining for pitting edema, you press gently inward on the swollen area with a finger for a few seconds. You then remove your finger. If the indentation remains and does not immediately disappear, that is pitting edema.

If there is pitting edema of the ankles, does the pitting edema extend up the lower leg. If it extends up the lower leg, does it extend up to the tibial plateau. I have seen bilateral pitting edema sometimes extending to the tibial plateau in my orthopedic office with some frequency. This is usually due to uncontrolled congestive heart failure. I call the internist or cardiologist and refer the patient directly to their office for evaluation and treatment of the uncontrolled congestive heart failure. Even though the patient is not seeing me with complaints of swollen ankles, proper medical care involves getting immediate proper medical care for the uncontrolled congestive heart failure.

Observation, observation, observation. It does not matter why the patient is seeing you in your office or place of work. Part of your initial evaluation should be a quick check of the ankles for swelling. It does not matter why the patient is seeing you in your office or place of work. If you see swelling of the ankles, examine for pitting edema. It does not matter why the patient is seeing you in your office or place of work. If you find pitting edema, spend the time to arrange for the patient to be seen and treated by the patient's medical provider expeditiously. Sorry. I am being preachy again.

Unilateral swelling involving much of the leg may be chronic lymphedema. It is important to note this since this diagnosis may be a contraindication to surgery on this leg.

In my initial observation, I check for hair growth on the toes. I find this is a quick check for adequate blood supply to the legs. If there is hair growth on the toes, then blood supply to this leg is probably satisfactory. With poor blood supply to the leg, one of the first "symptoms" is lack of hair growth on the toes. Press on the big toe and release to check capillary refill. Normally it takes less than three seconds for the vascularity to restore the color to the toe. More than three seconds raises concerns regarding decreased vascularity to the leg and foot.

Black areas at the tips of the toes suggests necrosis from the microvascular disease of diabetes mellitus or severe atherosclerotic peripheral vascular disease. All diabetics need to have their feet checked at every office visit. A free clinic I work at has signs on the wall stating, "Remove shoes and socks for every diabetic visit."

If there is unilateral swelling (i.e. one ankle, not both) is the swelling on one side of the ankle or both. Swelling on one side of the ankle may indicate a simple sprain of the deltoid or the lateral collateral ligaments. Swelling on one side may also indicate a soft tissue mass, often a lipoma or ganglion.

Does the leg and ankle have skin changes consistent with chronic venous stasis disease? Are there ulcers? Is there is globular type swelling equal medially and laterally? This may indicate an effusion of the ankle joint from inflammatory arthritis or infection.

For my palpation protocol, I gently palpate the medial malleolus, the deltoid ligament, the lateral malleolus and the lateral collateral ligaments. Tenderness in these areas may indicate fractures or sprains. I palpate the medial mid foot looking for a possible accessory navicular bone. I palpate the base of the fifth metatarsal looking for a possible fracture of the base of the fight metatarsal. If there are complaints of pain in a specific place, I palpate there looking for point tenderness which might indicate a fracture or calcific tendinitis. I palpate between the metatarsal heads looking for evidence of a Morton's neuroma. I palpate the metatarsal heads looking for evidence of metatarsalgia. I observe the first metatarsal phalangeal joint looking for a possible bunion and to evaluate its severity. I palpate the medial aspect of the first metatarsal phalangeal joint looking for possible tenderness. I palpate the sesamoid bones of the big toe looking for evidence of sesamoiditis. I move the first metatarsal joint up and down looking for pain on motion. Pain on motion of the first metatarsal phalangeal joint may be caused by gout or degenerative arthritis of that joint, called hallux rigidus. If the range of motion of the first metatarsal phalangeal joint is restricted then the diagnosis is more likely hallux rigidus.

I ask the patient to dorsiflex, plantar flex, invert and evert the ankle joint actively. If there is limitation of active motion, I check passive motion in each of the four directions.

I tap over the tarsal tunnel to perform a Tinel's sign test of the tibial nerve as it runs through the tarsal tunnel. This is important if the patient is complaining of medial ankle or foot pain. I have the patient evert the ankle while palpating at the lateral malleolus looking for subluxation of the peroneal tendons. This is important if the patient is complaining of lateral ankle or foot pain.

Deformities obvious to an initial glance may include a prominence at the middle of the medial mid foot. In a young person with medial foot pain, this may indicate the presence of a painful accessory navicular bone. An unusually high arch particularly with clawed toes suggests possible Charcot Marie Tooth disease. The degree of bunion, i.e. hallux valgus, can be determined from a glance. Similarly, look for hammer toes, overlapping toes and other deformities.

Have your patient stand on the floor or the step stool a patient uses to step up on to the examining table. From the front does the forefoot splay out in a pronated position. Place your fingers at the arch. Is there an arch present? Is no arch present? Does this patient have a flexible pronated flatfoot? Have the patient turn around and examine the heel from the back. Is the calcaneus positioned straight up and down? Does the heel angulate so that the calcaneus angles outward as it reaches the floor? Does the patient have calcaneal valgus?

Grasp the heel with one hand and the forefoot with the other. Try to move the forefoot left and right, i.e. medially and laterally on the calcaneus. There should be a small amount of painless motion when performing this maneuver. Rigidity may be due to old injury, degenerative arthritis or previous fusion surgery. In a young patient rigidity may be due to a tarsal coalition, in which a joint or joints have not formed properly and there are abnormal connections between one or more bones. This may be a cause of foot pain in a young person.

Pressure between the metatarsal heads using your thumb and middle finger may elicit pain in some patients. Particularly between the third and fourth metatarsal heads tenderness is consistent with a Morton's neuroma. Palpation of the metatarsal heads may indicate metatarsalgia if painful. Palpation of the metatarsal heads at the first metatarsal phalangeal joint if painful may indicate sesamoiditis.

# CHAPTER TWENTY THREE

# Documenting Your Medical History and Physical Examination

## The Perils of Copy and Paste in Electronic Medical Records

You have just completed a complex medical history and physical examination. What happens next? You have to document this information so that this information is accessible to other medical providers. I wish to discuss your documentation of that medical history and physical examination, which you just finished. If it is early morning and you are busy and rushed and wait until evening to document your history and physical examination, you will forget important details, you will omit important information, you will document your encounter with your patient in an abbreviated form, you will document your encounter with your patient inadequately. Yes, you will click on enough items to reach your preferred encounter level, but you will not remember or bother to document subtleties.

*Case Study:*
*Two quotes from two medical records, I recently reviewed when I saw the patients on referral, regarding the physical examination of a shoulder:*

*First quote: "full direction of motion"*

*Second quote: "the shoulder was non tender."*

What if any information is imparted by the statement that the shoulder had "full direction of motion." Do we really believe that the range of motion was tested in all directions and was full? I don't think so! The phrase, "full direction of motion," is meaningless. The use of that phrase indicates a lack of clear and logical thinking.

What if any information is imparted by the statement that the shoulder was non tender? Do we really believe that the examining physician carefully and thoroughly palpated each and every important anatomic structure of the shoulder? I don't think so! The phrase, the shoulder was non tender," really is meaningless. I intuit that at most, at best, the examining physician performed some casual, non specific stroking of the shoulder, somewhere about the shoulder and that the non specific stroking did not hurt.

**If the description of the medical history is not detailed and thorough, if the description of the physical examination is not detailed and thorough, you should assume that neither the actual medical history nor the actual physical examination were detailed and thorough.**

When you document your encounter with a patient, particularly with inpatients, it is important to elaborate on your thinking when recording your impression. If you go off call, you want whoever is covering for you to be able to quickly get a sense of what you were thinking and why and what you were planning.

I recall the first time that I picked up a several inch thick medical record (before electronic medical records). I was astounded and horrified at how opaque the medical record was. It took hours or would have taken hours to extract details from that record. Electronic medical records are even worse. With a paper chart you could flip through pages faster than you can skim the pages of an electronic record.

When you describe something, describe it so that someone reading your description will be able to draw or act out what you have described with accuracy. Unfortunately, our primary, secondary and tertiary education does not teach us to learn and perfect these skills. You will have to nurture these skills on your own.

I was fortunate in my Introduction to the Clinic course at Harvard Medical School to alight in a six week one on one mentor-tutee relationship with an outstanding physician and mentor, Herman Godwin, at Boston City Hospital in the summer of 1969. For six weeks, each morning I was assigned a patient. I, then, took as detailed a medical history as I was able to and performed as detailed physical examination as I was able to.

Every afternoon, Dr. Godwin, grilled me on speaking and writing clearly, concisely, accurately and thoroughly for whichever patient I was assigned that morning. Dr. Godwin would ask me to give the 30 second oral synopsis you might use when going off call. Then, he would ask for the three minute presentation you would give to a chief resident the morning after a patient was admitted. Then, the five minute presentation you might give at grand rounds to a visiting professor. Dr. Godwin also pushed me toward making my writing more clear, more concise, more logical and more thorough. Most medical provider trainees are not as fortunate as I was in obtaining this experience. You will need to work on this yourself.

When writing your impression of a patient in a chart, explain in detail what you are thinking and considering regarding possible diagnoses and possible treatments so that a medical provider taking over will not have to play catch up. You want the person taking over the care of your patient to be able to do so seamlessly.

As you go through your training, read the medical records written by other medical providers critically regarding the question, "Was the medical history and physical examination performed in sufficient detail and recorded in sufficient detail to allow you to truly visualize and understand what happened during each medical provider/patient encounter."

Documenting the patient's description of pain

Let's move on to descriptions of pain in medical records. Many perhaps most descriptions of pain in the medical records reference something like, "The patient complained of pain in the shoulder" or more abbreviated "pain in shoulder." Does this limited description of the shoulder pain give you much useful information? Does this limited description of the shoulder pain give you any useful information? I don't think so. Recently, I saw a patient referred with shoulder pain. The total description in the chart from the previous medical provider was "left shoulder pain."

Here is my description of this patient's shoulder pain following my history taking of his complaint and demonstration of radiation of the pain, when I asked, "Does the pain travel anywhere else." "Patient complains of pain in the anterior left shoulder radiating mostly to the left upper arm, but also, at times, down the forearm and into the ring and little finger." Reading the initial description, you would focus only on the shoulder. Taking a careful medical history and then describing the patient's "actual" pain leads to a more thoughtful and extensive evaluation. Thinking about and describing the patient's "actual" pain in detail leads to the recognition that this patient may have more than one diagnosis. The differential diagnosis list of possible diagnoses for this patient following my detailed description of his pain expands to include herniated cervical disc with pain radiating into the T1 dermatome, cubital tunnel syndrome and other ulnar nerve problems causing pain radiating into the ring and little finger as well as an intrinsic shoulder problem.

In order to communicate detailed, complete and accurate information about the patient's pain or discomfort, you first have to take a detailed, complete and accurate history. Have the patient describe the pain, discomfort or unpleasant sensation. Is it sharp and acute in nature? Diffuse? Achy? Crampy? Does it stay in one place? Does it travel? If so, where does it travel to? Is the pain or discomfort steady? Does it come and go? If so how often? How severe does the pain become? Have you ever had any pain like this before? How does the discomfort interfere with activities or sleep? Then record all of that in the medical record.

Back to observation. Watching a patient move his hands while attempting to describe his patient is often revealing.

Describing the palpation exam

In order to report a detailed, accurate and complete "palpation" part of the examination of some part of the body, you first have to perform a detailed and complete palpation examination of that part of the body. You need to specify which structures you palpated. Thus, for example, for the shoulder: "The sterno-clavicular joint, the clavicle, the acromio-clavicular joint, the biceps tendon and the point of the shoulder were non tender to palpation." Or, for the knee: "The patella, the medial collateral ligament, the medial knee joint line, the pes anserinus bursa and the tibial tubercle were not tender. The lateral collateral ligament was tender at the origin."

Similarly, a description of the palpation of a mass should include location, size, firmness, smoothness or irregularity, texture or consistency, fixation or moveability and so on. In order for the description of a mass to be this detailed, it requires, of course, that the physical examination be sufficiently thoughtful and thorough to include evaluation of all of these characteristics of a mass. For example, "There was an irregular mass approximately 5 cm by 2 cm on the dorsal radial aspect of the hand in line with the index finger. The mass had a woody consistency." This description allows you to "see" and "feel" the mass in a second hand way. This description allows you to understand that this mass may be an infection with mycobacterium marinum.

Describing the breast exam

For a description of a breast exam, the chart may reflect, "Breast exam normal." How much confidence do you have that the examining medical provider performed a complete and thorough exam? Contrast the description of a breast exam above with this description, "A complete breast examination of both breasts including all four quadrants with light, medium and deep pressure was performed. No nodules or tenderness was noted. There was no nipple discharge." Or, if a nodule was detected: "A 3 mm nodule was noted in the right upper quadrant of the right breast. It was slightly tender to deep palpation, had a firm consistency and was easily moveable." You can picture this nodule and the physical examination of this nodule.

Describing Motion

Consider this description, "The shoulder had full motion." Do you have confidence that the examining medical provider actually, carefully tested all of the ranges of motion of the shoulder? I don't. Consider this description, "Right shoulder active motion: forward flexion 60 degrees, extension 30 degrees, abduction 70 degrees, internal rotation 20 degrees, external rotation 40 degrees." This is a clear description of a patient with a frozen shoulder. You, the reader, can visualize the actual examination of active motion of that shoulder. You know a careful active range of motion examination was performed.

At times it is important to document that there is a difference between active motion and passive motion. For example, a patient with rheumatoid arthritis and a drooping ring and little finger. Documenting that there is full passive extension of the metacarpal phalangeal joints with absence of active extension clearly describes and documents the physical examination of a patient with rupture of the extensor tendons to the ring and little fingers. You can mentally visualize the physical examination of the hand based on that description.

Describing fractures on x-rays

Only rare emergency room physicians are able to describe an x-ray of a fracture to me in such a way that I am able to draw a picture of the x-ray. Granted this was more important before the era of the mobile phone and access to x-rays on line. The ER doc now takes a picture and emails it to the covering physician. Now the covering physician signs into the hospital system on line and looks up the x-ray. Your description should include which bone is or bones are broken. Also, which part or parts of the bone are broken. For example, the head, neck subtrochanteric area, mid shaft, distal metaphysis and condyles of the femur.

Your description should include information regarding whether there are two, three or multiple fragments of bone. Is the joint dislocated? Are the fracture fragments non displaced, minimally displaced, one quarter inch displaced or widely displaced? Thus, a description may be: "I see a fracture of the proximal femur with three large fragments. There is more than half an inch displacement. The femoral head is dislocated from the acetabulum and displaced proximally." You are able to draw an approximate picture of the fracture dislocation of the hip from this description.

Or this description: "The x-rays of the forearm of this seven year old girl show that both the radius and the ulnar shafts are bent about twenty degrees. I do not see a fracture line on x-ray." This is a sufficiently accurate description of greenstick fractures of both bones of the forearm.

Electronic Medical Records

Many electronic medical record (EMR) systems are designed so that you point and click your physical examination. This allows the EMR system to automatically determine a level of complexity of the exam for billing purposes. I have seen systems which alert the medical provider to the fact that the physical examination is not complete enough to allow a higher level of billing. This encourages the medical provider to add unnecessary parts of the physical examination to allow for higher billing.

These "point and click" systems deter and inhibit the habits of entering a complete and complex history and physical examination. A major issue with the use of EMR systems is the fact that entering data into a computer by a human being is time consuming and laborious. This tends to deter and inhibit the habits of entering detailed and complete information. I am hopeful that the evolution of EMR systems will reach the point at which data may be entered quickly and effortlessly by voice alone. At such a time it will be easier to document in detail the medical history and physical examination. The current problem is the fact that if you are not going to enter detailed information into the EMR system, you are not going to bother obtaining that information when you perform your physical examination. The result will be inferior and limited medical histories and inferior and limited physical examinations.

The Uses and Abuses of Copy and Paste in Electronic Medical Records

When seeing a patient for follow up, it is easy, it is effortless, it is smooth, it is efficient, it seems natural and good to copy and paste some or all of the previous record, when documenting the current medical provider/patient interaction.

*Case Study:*

*I am referred a patient by an insurance company and asked to perform an independent medical evaluation on a patient who alleged injury a year and three months previously. The insurance company provides the medical records of the treating medical provider covering the fifteen month period of treatment. The medical provider has seen this patient monthly since the injury. The medical record covers the initial office visit and the fourteen follow up visits.*

*I review the print out of the electronic medical records. For the fourteen follow up visits, the medical records are "identical". By "identical," I mean, "identical." When I look up the definition of "identical" online I read, "similar in every detail, exactly alike." Yes, I mean "identical." For each follow up visit, the medical provider clearly copied and pasted the previous visit without the slightest alteration. Even the punctuation and spacing were the same.*

*In my report to the insurance company, I stated that the medical record was worthless in trying to determine what actually happened during the previous fourteen months. This lack of accurate recording of medical history and physical examination information harmed the patient's ability to claim continuing problems. This is a true story.*

The above case study is obviously an egregious and fraudulent use of the copy and paste function. I have seen identical medical records on numerous other occasions. This is lazy behavior. This is fraudulent behavior. This is stupid behavior. I think I am preaching again. Enough said.

*Case Study:*

*I receive a medical record from a professor of medicine at a major medical center. In the interval history section, there has clearly been copy, paste and edit behavior. Most but not all of the details of this section have been edited correctly to reflect the new information. Two sentences which reflect the patient stopped a specific medication two months ago is incorrect. This information was correct when the patient was first seen 18 months previously. It is not correct when repeated 18 months later.*

A small error you say. I agree. It does seem a small error. From the small acorns of error, large oak trees of harm may grow. My point. This professor of medicine was doing a careful job of documenting the follow up visit. Yet, even with care, the error "snuck in" because of the use of copy and paste which is efficient and time saving. In my career I saw a steady stream of copy and paste errors which occurred when the medical provider used copy and paste to bring information forward.

**The easy and frequent use of copy and paste in the use of electronic medical records has allowed frequent errors in documenting the medical history and in documenting the physical exam to occur.**

**Beware: Do not allow the use of copy and paste in electronic medical records lure you into sloppy and inaccurate documentation of your medical histories and physical examinations.**

# CHAPTER TWENTY FOUR:

# Coda

---

I have reached the denouement of my efforts to instruct and yes harangue you toward excellence in practice of medicine. Excellence in the practice of medicine requires excellence in each small part of medicine: excellence in attitude, excellence in logical thinking, excellence in medical history taking, excellence in physical examination performance, excellence in thoughtful analysis, excellence in decision making, excellence in actions such as surgery and excellence in providing compassion and counseling to your patients. The underlying issue is attitude and the continuing attempt to strive for excellence in all aspects of the practice of medicine.

My sermon is complete.

Enjoy your learning of the practice of clinical medicine.

Enjoy your actual practice of clinical medicine.

I hope I have provided some limited positive influence on your medical career.

Be well. Live long and prosper. God spede you well!